Advanced Methods of Weight Training

(Original Version, Restored)

by

BOB HOFFMAN

Olympic Coach

Originally published in 1951

PUBLISHED BY O'Faolain Patriot L L C, Copyright 2012

info@physicalculturebooks.com

ISBN-13: 978-1470161392

ISBN-10: 1470161397

Published in the United States of America

To Order More Copies Visit:
PhysicalCultureBooks.com

appropriate for the reader's needs or expectations. The publisher expressly disclaims any and all responsibility and/or liabilities that might result from the uninformed or misinformed application of the techniques identified herein as well as for any unsupervised physical fitness training.

Finally, the publisher disclaims any and all liabilities arising from the use of any equipment featured in this book and makes no representations as to the utility, safety, or adequacy of the equipment generally or with respect to any specific purpose.

York Advanced Methods of Weight Training

All kinds of people take up the practice of weight training. The majority are those who wish to keep fit in the easiest and quickest manner. Fortunately for them keeping fit with weights requires little time and effort, only reasonable persistence with a weight training course such as Bob Hoffman's Simplified System of Barbell Training, to be twice as strong as the average man, to be well enough built to attract favorable attention in street clothes or at the beach, to enjoy splendid health, to have good endurance, rapid recuperative power and the expectancy of long life. There are a great many who use weights to overcome the ravages of ill health, to build a weak, sickly body to strength and health, there are those who desire to rejuvenate an injured limb or other part of the body, a fair number who wish to reduce their overweight bodies, to replace ugly fat with smooth, strong muscles, a great many who wish to gain weight, to build their undeveloped frames so that they will compare favorably with the advanced barbell men.

There are many who train with weights to improve their athletic ability, to develop more speed, power, nervous energy or super endurance so that they can perform better at their chosen sport. Weight lifting will improve any man at his favorite sport and a great many of the nations top athletes, national champions and record holders, are weight trained men. There are others who desire to be weight lifting champions, to make the world's championship and Olympic teams, there are many who desire to be strong, to be the strongest man in their district, there are even more who want to pack all the muscle they can upon their frames, and last, but far from least, there is the large group who find pleasure, satisfaction and fame, which can result in time in fortune, by building such a magnificent physique that they will be winners in physique contests, perhaps "Mr. America" or even obtain the greatest prize of all, "Mr. Universe" or "Mr. World."

If all you want is to keep fit in the easiest possible way you can do this with the simplified course contained in this group of courses in a few minutes a day, three or four times a week, lifting only moderate poundages. Most of the other types of barbell men enumerated, will obtain all they desire in a physical way from the Four Famous York Courses which have developed more champions of strength and development, more lifting champions, more physique champions, than all other courses combined. Those who desire athletic improvement will succeed best by following the exercises of the Four York Courses, with particular emphasis on the weight lifting courses. Although this course can be used by any man who is not a complete beginner at weight training, it is primarily designed for the man who desires the limit in muscle, in strength and development. For the man who wants big, strong muscles in the right places so that he will have perfect proportions, the man who may wish to enter physique contests and win great honors and then go on to teaching others by running a gymnasium of his own.

The author of this group of courses has already sold more than a million other courses and books of which he is the author, he is the editor of Strength & Health magazine, the world's largest selling body building magazine. He is the Olympic coach and has developed hundreds of champions of strength and development. His York Barbell Club Team have been U.S. lifting champions every year since 1932, have been world's champions since 1937, year after year the teams he coaches and trains win the world's weight lifting titles. All but one or two of the official Mr. America's are York trained men, most of them members of the York Barbell Club. The four "Mr. Universes" to date, all Americans, John Grimek, Steve Stanko, Steeve Reeves and John Farbotnik, trained at York before winning their greatest triumph. Over a period of years, the author of this course has come to be known as "The Builder of Champions," "The World's Greatest Weight Lifting Coach." He is well qualified to help you obtain the limit in strength and development as he has already done for so many others.

York courses which have long been included with York weight training sets are still the best for the particular purpose for which they were designed. It is not our intention to replace anyone of them with this course. It has been our attempt to offer the most complete barbell training treatise ever compiled. A Book which supplies definite training schedules, which offers you the exact schedules so many of the greats of the present have used. It supplies you with their methods of training and of living. You can be sure when you follow the courses and training advice offered in these pages that you are following THE BEST WAY, for no other instructor, no other group of instructors, can match the magnitude of our successes, no other club or individual coach has produced so many champions.

By following this complete book of courses exactly as it is written, following the training advice offered, your success is assured. This is the most complete treatise, the most scientific group of courses on weight training, ever compiled. It provides you with the best instruction and the most successful methods.

The group of courses contained in this treatise has been designed primarily for the advanced body builder, the man who has already made considerable progress in building his body, the man who wishes to go on in building the finest possible physique, the most muscle, to gain fame for his physique, to have his picture on the cover of Strength & Health magazine, and to teach others. It should not be necessary to explain every little training detail, as the men who use this course will have had experience, but we do wish to offer these few reminders which must be observed to obtain the best results in the shortest time.

1.   To succeed, never miss an exercise period. If due to unavoidable circumstances, you are forced to miss a period, make up for

it or you will find it easier to miss in the future. Be sure you don't offer yourself excuses, regularity is a major essential of success. Missing your training is a retarding factor which will lead to ultimate failure in the end. If you train Monday, Wednesday, and Friday and are forced to miss your training on Wednesday for instance, exercise on Thursday and Saturday, or two days in succession if that is more convenient.

2.   Keep yourself warm while exercising. Wear sweat clothes or other warm clothing when training, except when you are in the hot summer sun, keep out of drafts.

The Best Time to Train

3.   Is after the days work is done, with enough time before the evening meal to permit an hour before dining. The famous members of the York Barbell Club train at 4 P.M. If you exercise in the evening be sure that it is an hour or two after your meal, allowing enough time before retiring for an hour of reading or relaxing.

4.   Muscular size and shape is gained by a combination of proper exercise, adequate nourishment and rest.

5. Be sure that your diet includes enough of the protective foods, milk, cheese, and other dairy products, eggs, fresh meat, some of an organic nature such as liver, heart, kidneys, etc., plenty of green and yellow vegetables, leafy vegetables and fruits of all sorts. When your diet includes the protective foods, you can eat anything else you like, which likes you.

6. 8 hours of sleep is sufficient for the average. Many find 6 enough, and younger, growing, hard training men, need as much as 10 hours. If you get up in the morning feeling "like a million," you will know that you are getting enough sleep.

7. To lose weight reduce the amount of sugars, starches and fats which you consume. Don't eliminate them entirely, for your body needs a certain amount of these foods, but too much of a good thing, coupled with a sedentary life is what causes the fat to pile on.

8. To gain weight eat plenty of good, wholesome food, thick soups, solid vegetables, a quart of milk at least each day, plenty of protein foods, the material of which the body is made, soy beans in various forms are excellent, nuts are weight producing and nourishing. If you are young and very active you can eat snacks between meals at regular

intervals. Lying down before and after meals will help you gain weight. Eat under happy, harmonious conditions, if you are upset mentally do not eat at that time. Masticate your food well and digestion and assimilation will be easier.

9.   A lukewarm bath is best, little more than body temperature. Hot baths are tiring, devitalizing, make one sleepy. Cold baths are a shock to the system, if you like them there is no harm in them.

10.   A rub down after a good workout has it's advantages. Hoffman's rub, diluted with 2 ounces of the rub to a pint of water, or alcohol is ideal for this purpose. Apply full strength for aches or pains, strains or sprains.

11.   After a workout take a good shower, then a rub, if possible lay down for a time. This part of the training is very important.

12.   It is most beneficial if you perform the movements of your exercises with moderate slowness so that the weight resistance can be felt every inch of the way, almost as much benefit is obtained in lowering as in raising the weight,

13.   Each exercise should be performed over the longest possible range, from the

extreme of contraction to the limit of extension.

It's Important to Breathe Properly

14.   It's important to breathe as much and as deeply as necessary. Usually inhalation takes place during the hardest half of the exercise, exhalation as the weight is lowered.

15.   You are sure to register satisfactory gains by training progressively with weights as outlined in this book, providing you follow the major rules of health. Obtain sufficient sleep, rest and relaxation, maintain a tranquil mind, eat a wide variety of good food at meal times only and obtain a good share of fresh air and sunlight.

16.   The chief benefit derived from weight training is the stimulation of the internal works of the body. Speeded up respiration and circulation assure that the blood will be properly oxygenized so that each cell received its share of oxygen and glycogen or blood sugar, and the waste products of combustion are removed. To insure that the body is obtaining plenty of oxygen walk around between exercises and breathe deeply. It is the habit of the author of this book to walk around and take 25 to 30 deep breaths between exercises. This walking about and

deep breathing has become generally known as the Hoffman Walk, and should be an important part of your training.

17.   We have suggested that you keep yourself warm while exercising where it is cool and there are drafts, but if you are training in a warm room or in the sun on a warm day, you should wear as little as possible. Perspiration is always beneficial and the alchemy of the sun's ray is a great aid in health and muscle building.

18.   Although you must constantly strive to handle more and more weight, you should not work on your nerve too often. Except on your limit day of training, you should train well within your capabilities, in other words train, but do not strain.

19.   Warming up is most important, it means to start the blood circulating vigorously through the muscles before exercising strenuously. By warming the muscles in this manner, possibilities of strains and sprains is eliminated. It is not wise to suddenly stop exercising at the completion of a very hard exercise, better to taper off with a few moderate exercises before discontinuing training.

20.   There are so many pieces of good, result producing, health and muscle building apparatus, that it is not possible to use them all in one tinkering day a week. Therefore it is wise to have two tinkering days each week, if possible. The various muscle building appliances, expanders, health shoes, giant crusher grip, wrist roller, pulleys, head strap, etc., are a pleasure to use, develop the muscles from many different angles and build a really outstanding physique.

21.   The regular York courses with their 11 barbell exercises and 7 dumbell exercises will suffice for any beginner, but advanced men can practice more exercises as they develop the ability to keep going, to practice a great many more exercises. The most ambitious trainees follow at least two complete courses of 12 exercises each, or the equivalent in set training. There are some men who can do more, practice each exercise three times or 36 exercises in all. Some practice their favorite exercises five times and thus have a workout of at least 40 exercises. Only you know how much you can do and still make gains, this must be determined by the progress you make and how you feel.

How To Use The York Bar Bell Courses

22.   While each York course differs to some extent from others, all are designed so that all the major muscle groups of the body receive a fair share of work. Regardless of your ambitions or desires in physical training, you should always practice at least one of the well planned, scientifically arranged York courses before going on to any type of specialization. After you have performed the essentials, followed any complete York course, preferably one of the barbell courses, you can proceed as you desire with the assurance that satisfactory physical gains are sure to result.

23.   Moderate days of training. This subject has been covered to a fair degree under the heading, "tinkering" days. There should always be some moderate days of training. Days on which the muscles are given a nice, comfortable, stimulating workout, a workout which tones the muscles, and prepares them for the harder training days to come. The moderate exercises develop the muscles from different angles, stretch them, keeping the body loose, flexible and athletic.

24.   Perform the exercises correctly. Each exercise is designed to develop some particular muscle or group of muscles. If you do not perform these exercises correctly, instead of being a good exercise for that part of the body for which it is intended, it will be a poor exercise for several parts of the body. For instance, if you are performing the two hands curl, and you "cheat," the back will be brought into action and the weights swung to the upper chest. On most training days perform all exercises correctly, steadily, while exerting maximum force and return to the starting position with comparative slowness. Only on the limit day of training is some "cheating" permitted.

The Amount of Weight to Use

25.   It is difficult to tell any man just how much weight to use for ambitious barbell men vary so much in size, strength, quality of muscle, muscular leverage, ambition, willingness to work and endurance, that every man must be his own trainer to a degree, for only he knows ho he feels, only he knows what he wants and how much he can do. The man using this course should have trained enough to know what weights he can handle correctly and for how many repetitions. One must select only enough

weight in the first movements to make possible the satisfactory conclusion of the program. You should select the amount of weight which you can correctly handle for the scheduled number of repetitions and still complete your training program without working on your nerve more than once per week.

26.   The Breathing squat, is very popular in most weight training circles. The vigorous use of the largest and strongest muscles of the body, those of the legs and hips, demand a great deal of nutriment. The heart and lung action is greatly amplified when they are placed in vigorous use. When this exertion is felt, breathing is greatly increased, but it is a physiological fact that additional oxygen must be absorbed only as the demand is created. Therefore breathing squats which schedule five deep breaths between movements are of little benefit in the beginning. I recommend single breaths until the need is created, then 2, 3 or 5 as required. A good plan with a very heavy weight is to take one breath the first bend, two the second, three the third, four the fourth, five the fifth and then continue with this number.

27.   Constantly strive to handle more and more weight. Progression is the only way to

succeed in building your body. We do not stand still in this life, we go either forward or back. And your success will be governed by your ability to go forward, to improve. You must constantly strive to overcome greater resistance, for only by making increasing demands with the necessary rest days intervening, can you attain your physical desires.

28.   Water, milk or fruit juice are being consumed in some quarters in large quantities during training. This rather popular practice is not a good habit, particularly for the beginner or the man of limited experience. It will harm the advanced barbell man less, for his inner works are tough and durable and will stand a lot of misuse and abuse. As it is wise to refrain from eating just before or right after training, it is not wise to take liquid food at the same time or during the training, for milk and fruit juices are liquid food. There is ample opportunity to consume enough milk and juices at regular meal times or snacks between meals when you are not training. The object of taking liquids during training is to gain weight. It is estimated that three fourths of the body is liquid, naturally imbibing more liquid will temporarily mean more weight, but liquid is not muscle, fat is

made up largely of liquid, so too many body builders who drink excess quantities of milk get fat. You don't want that kind of increased weight, you should desire a well proportioned, strong and attractive body.

29.   Salt tabs. Profuse perspiration is good for you, that's one of the reasons we recommend that you keep yourself warm during cool or cold weather when training, and we want you to train in the sun when conditions permit. Perspiration cleans the pores and greatly aids the organs of elimination. With the perspiration, many of the essential salts of the body are lost and should be replaced with salt tabs. You can obtain them at any drug store. Drink only enough water during training, if you must drink, to replace the moisture lost through perspiration.

Know Your Muscles

30.   While it is not necessary that you study the anatomy of the body thoroughly, it is wise to know the name, location and action of the muscles of the body. You will find the names and location of the muscles on the charts which are a part of a number of York courses. When your periodic inspections before a mirror, indicate that some part of

your body is not responding to training as you desire, you can select exercises designed to develop these particular muscles.

31.   Set a goal. You must set a goal, a desire to become stronger, to gain more muscle, to build an admiration creating physique, to improve your health, to overcome your deficiencies, to be a champion weight lifter or a physique contest winner, to be Mr. America. This setting of a goal, may be called hitching your ambition to a star. but first you must know what you want, then you must have the willingness to work hard, long and intelligently toward that goal. Don't let anything prevent your success.

32.   Getting bell on chest for bench press. If you are training with one or more companions, the simplest way to get a bell in position for a heavy bench press, is to have your training partner help you place it there. If you are training alone, the easiest way is to have a pair of supports a bit higher than your head, to hold the bell, slide under the bell, lift it off and perform the necessary movements. Some men clean the bell to the shoulders, sit on the bench and then rock or roll back into the starting position. If the weight is heavier, you can pull it to your thighs, sit down, roll it to the top of the thighs, then to the abdomen,

and with a belly toss and the help of the hands and arms, get it into the pressing position. If you become good at the pull over and press you can pull your weight over in that way.

33.   Leg Pressing Machine. The leg press is a good exercise, but most men unassisted can not place a heavy enough weight upon their feet. A strong man as an exercise, can leg press 400 or 500 pounds. Even if he can get this amount of weight on his legs it is dangerous and difficult to control. That is why the author of this course designed a popular leg press machine, which permits the use of very heavy weights without strain or danger, as it eliminates all hazard, and provides ease of handling the weight. Such a machine is part of every commercial or public gym and should be a part of every home gym.

34.   There are men who have performed repetition deep knee bends with 500 pounds, yet no man can get this amount of weight on the shoulders unassisted. To advance to a limit poundage in the deep knee bend you need training partners to help you get the weight on your shoulders or better still you should have a deep knee bend stand. York offers a pair of these stands at a moderate

cost which will make it possible for anyone to use heavy weights in this exercise and the use of heavy weights is the only successful method to obtain a full measure of benefit from this exercise. A pair of deep knee bend stands should be a part of every home gymnasium.

35.   The 5 in 1 Muscle Builder is another contribution to the strength, health and muscle seeking public by the author of this book of courses. The 5 in 1 Muscle Builder occupies no more space than a large chair, is not higher than a normal door, yet it is 5 machines in one. It includes a strong bench, for bench work of all sorts, an incline bench which can also be used as a decline bench making possible the practice of a great many excellent and result producing exercises, which in many cases are comparatively new and little known. It includes an abdominal board which is an essential in every home. The machine is made to be a strong barbell rack. And one of the finest features is the overhead pulley which is a part of this machine. Pulley weights have been used with splendid effect by most of the physique contest stars. They build, impressive, nice to look at muscles, with very little effort. The 5

in 1 Muscle Builder should be a part of every home gym.

Keep A Record

36.   With a training record you will know just what exercises you have performed each training day, and a study of this record will indicate whether you have been neglecting some muscles or getting into training ruts, performing the same exercise too often. You will succeed better if you put your whole heart, soul and body back of your strength, health and muscle building program. Make a science of your physical improvement schedule, and you can't do this if you don't keep records to indicate what you have been doing, recording the progress of lack of progress you are making.

37.   Circulation improving movements. The chief benefit derived from physical training is the speeding up of the circulation. This assures that all parts of the body, each of the estimated 3 trillion cells, will obtain a full measure of nutriment. Sluggish circulation results in internal inefficiency, a toxic condition of the blood, fatigue and later diseases and death. You youthify, liven and improve every internal process by practicing exercises which amplify the circulation and

active all internal organs and glands. Those exercises which put into action the largest and strongest muscles of the body, those farthest from the heart, exercises which utilize all the muscles and those which activate the mid section are most beneficial. For these latter exercises in particular, strengthen, squeeze, massage and amplify the action of all organs and glands, all internal processes. They improve respiration, assimilation and elimination. As the muscles on the outside of the body are strengthened, your internal organs and glands, become more prolific and stronger in their actions.

38.   You get out of exercise what you put into it. You pay for what you get in this world. Pay a little, get a little, pay more, get more. And by paying in physical training, we mean more training, harder training, a closer adherence to the rules of right living. If you ambition is great, to realize it, your effort must be great. The effort expended is very little considering the great reward you obtain for your efforts, your improved appearance, better health, greater strength and more muscle. So plan to make maximum gains, plan to keep progressing, train hard and long and excellent results are sure to accrue.

39.   Your exertion can easily be measured by your puffing, panting and perspiring. The puffing and panting assures that your respiration has been speeded up, the perspiring, that you have been working vigorously to build up the heat which causes perspiration and aids in elimination.

40.   A Home Gymnasium or special training room, is a room which can be beneficially used by all the family, by father and mother, by the children, by the old folks too, for exercise is highly beneficial at any age. You can allot a room as a Home Gym and gradually you can equip it. Over a period of time, at nominal cost, using only the money which otherwise would be used for cigarettes, medicines, and doctor's bills, you can possess and profit from the use of every desirable piece of training equipment. In addition to a heavy set of weights, you need squat stands, leg press machine, 5 in 1 Muscle Builder, Expanders, Giant Crusher Grip, a lifting belt, etc. Place photos on the wall, have books and magazines on hand. A happy, strong and healthy family will result from the planning, equipping and the using of the Home Gym you should provide for yourself and family.

41.   Make a success story of your life. Exercising vigorously and progressively, scientifically, following the proven York and Bob Hoffman principles will make a success story of your life. You can have a body of which you will be proud, you will be super healthy and have a physique which will cause favorable remarks everywhere you go. In time, you may become a Strength & Health cover man. The best physical specimens today, were in most cases only average to begin, in many cases they were sick and ailing, and physically handicapped. By following the right methods, Bob Hoffman's methods, they reached the heights in the strength world. By following the same proven to be the best system, the method contained in this book of courses, you too can do as well.

42.   Superior results are obtained when the muscles are not worked in the same groove always, when a multitude of exercises are practiced over a period of time. To succeed best, you need considerable variety in your training, so particularly on the nights when you have more time, more energy, more ambition, when you feel like a million, take a real workout, consisting two or three courses as outlined in this book. By training

hard and following the Strength & Health system of living, you will gain rapidly.

43.   Be persistent. Don't offer excuses to yourself to miss an exercise period. Laziness is the most popular excuse for missing training, so don't let laziness get you. When you set a goal, when you persist, never deviate from your plan, your success will be in direct proportion to the effort you expend, and the health and efficiency of the body with which you are working, your own. So to succeed, be persistent, live right, eliminate entirely or cut to the barest minimum all harmful practices.

44.   Follow the rules of successful living. Your strength, your endurance, and your recuperative powers will quickly improve if you follow the rules of health. While a strong barbell man can stand more misuse and abuse of his body, it is not good for him either. Strong men can drink more, smoke more, do what they want more, because their efficient bodies will throw off poisons more rapidly than the bodies of average people. But why continue these habits which definitely are not good for you? Determine right now to eliminate them entirely. Very few men who reach the heights smoke or drink alcoholic beverages. Your instructor won many races

or contests in the last foot and with the last lift and as he never smoked or drank, as he closely followed the rules of right living, one thing sure this is an important reason for his success.

Don't Neglect Your Dumbell Training

45.   Although good results can be had with barbell training alone, although no exercise program is complete without barbells, the very best physiques invariably result from a great deal of moderate and heavy dumbbell training, coupled with barbell training. Heavy barbell work will build great power, bodyweight and big muscles but not the shapliness which results when both barbells and dumbbells are combined in a training program. So don't neglect your dumbbell training.

46.   Concentrate on the development of your muscles. The best results are not obtained if you work only by the clock, so much time, so much weight, so many repetitions. It would be better for you if you could, (few can) to forget the counts and continue until you are comfortably tired, not exhausted. In any event, think of the muscles which are involved in a particular exercise.

Make demands upon them, concentrate upon their development, tense them as they move in exercises and superior results will be obtained.

47.　　When the body is inactive most of the blood is in the organs, little of it is in the extremities; even during normal activity, only one sixth as much blood circulated below the ankles as above. When the blood is inactive, it transports little glycogen, less oxygen, the materials which are utilized to create exertion of any sort, but when a demand is created, great activity takes place within the body. Therefore, when one exercises vigorously with weights, particularly with exercises which involve all the muscles, great quantities of oxygen are carried by the blood, the body is thoroughly oxygenized, fatigue is eliminated as this thorough oxygenization of the blood is what eliminated fatigue, creates the feeling of well being, of feeling like a million, which all devotees of weight training report.

Why Some Succeed and Others Fail

48.　　Some few fail by training too hard, working too much on their nerve and not having a body which can back up this training, the desired gains are not made, more fail because they train too little, use weights which are too light, some fail because they follow the wrong system. The men in this latter class can succeed in a pleasing and satisfactory manner if they will follow the courses in this book exactly as they are written and of course follow the rules of healthful living also. But the majority of failures result because the body is unable to properly respond to the training. This can be the result of heredity, starting with a weak body, but more likely it is the mode of living. Change your ways and better results are sure to be gained. Poor nutrition is one of the chief causes of failure. Be sure that you receive your share of the protective foods which are mentioned elsewhere in this volume.

49.   How many training periods per week? In this book you will find the 3 times a week, the 5 times a week, and the 3! times a week schedules. With one vigorous training period per week, you should be able to keep in pretty good condition when once you reach that stage of development. With 2 training periods per week some progress should be made, with 3 training periods good progress, and with 4 training periods weekly, even more rapid progress. The best results will be

had with the 5 days a week training system described elsewhere in these pages.

50.   Details of each exercise are very important. We have endeavored to make the description of the various exercises as simple and as understandable as possible. There are frequently 3 or 4 apparently small details which must be understood and followed. Carefully read every word of the description of an exercise before attempting it, as your success depends upon the proper execution of the exercise. Read and study the courses at intervals. You will discover or rediscover some important training advice you have overlooked or not quite understood.

51.   There are two ways of holding the barbell. One the undergrip, which permits the bell to rest on the palms of the hands, as you raise the bell. There is the overgrip in which you grasp the bell with the knuckles up, the thumbs below. Then there is the reverse grip, the bar is held with the palms turned toward each other. In most exercises the bar is held with the hands at shoulder width apart, but various positions practiced at times will place the muscles in action in varying manners, with resulting benefit in muscle building. For instance, in the upright rowing motion, some perform the movement with the hands wide

apart, and at times with the hands only six inches apart. In most exercises the feet are held on the line a comfortable distance apart, about shoulder width, this aids balance. In some few movements such as the side to side bend, or the various toe raises, the heels may be held together. Except in the stiff legged dead weight lift and one or two other movements, the weight is lifted with a flat back. Throughout the course, this will be known as the starting position. The feet shoulder width apart, the hips low, the back flat, the head raised slightly, hands shoulder width apart, knuckles up.

Long Successful York Training Principles

It is not a happy accident that York men invariably win the greatest honors in strength and physique contests. The plain, simple and understandable fact is that York men have long followed the BEST WAY, the world's best system of weight training. A dozen books, a dozen courses, hundreds of magazine articles, have explained and taught the superior York or Bob Hoffman, training methods. The champions have learned, absorbed, and utilized these training methods, and that is why they are champions. It is our endeavor to compile in one moderate sized booklet, the essentials of the York System, in simple, understandable, readily useable form, so that any advanced barbell man can practically utilize this priceless instruction. Since volumes have been required to teach the complete story, you can appreciate that it is difficult to put the complete York training system in a single moderate sized volume, but we have done our best. One thing sure, never before has so much instruction, so many training secrets, so many courses, so many good exercises, so much living and training advice, so many methods of specialization and of advanced training been offered in a single volume.

Time Proven York Training Principles

1.   The Single Progressive System.

2.   The Double Progressive System.

3.   The Three Days a Week Training System.

4.   The Five Days a Week Training System.

5.   Irregular Training.

6.   Limited Programs.

7.   Other Schemes of Progression.

8.   The York Heavy and Light System.

9.   The Compound System.

10.   The York Set System.

11.   Upper and Lower Body Systems.

12.   Flushing the Muscles.

13.   Overload System.

14.   Specialization.

15.   The Thousand Exercises.

16.   Advanced Routines.

Of these advanced training methods, all but the single progressive, the three day a week and the limited program were originally and exclusively Bob Hoffman training principles. They have all been contained in the original York courses which have been offered to the strength and development seeking public for more than a score of years. We have lead in all phases of Body Building, others have followed.

The Single Progressive System

This method of training has served well for nearly a century. It is based on the principle that it is natures way to meet demands made upon the body, to train one day, rest the next. In using this system the body builder usually begins with 6 repetitions of a weight which he can correctly handle, rest the next day, then increase the repetitions to 7, rest a day, then 8, rest a day, then 9, etc., until the desired number of repetitions are attained, 10 to 15 as the particular exercise and your training desires will decree. When the maximum number of repetitions is reached, usually 12 to 15, add 5 pounds for upper body movements, 10 pounds for lower body movements, reduce the repetitions to 6, and start the single progressive system again. This type of training can be carried on for a considerable period.

The Double Progressive System

This is an original York principle and differs from the single progressive in the fact that it requires twice as long to progress with it and gives the body more time to become accustomed to the added work asked of it, more time for the important internal changes in organic and glandular action, which in time will result in the acquisition of a great deal more strength, muscle, super health and physical ability. Start with 6 movements as with the single progressive, rest a day, then practice 6 repetitions again, rest a day, then 7, rest a day, 7 again, continue in this manner until the desired maximum repetitions are attained, usually 12 to 15, add to the weight, reduce the counts to 6 and continue with the double progressive method. For those who are easy gainers, the Single Progressive System will at first suffice and when it becomes harder to gain, the double progressive can be employed. The double progressive system will serve best for those who are weaker than usual to begin, who are long out of training, who have been ill, or who for any other reason are unable to gain as fast as is demanded with the Single Progressive System.

The Three Days A Week Training System

With the three day a week training system, Monday, Wednesday and Friday are the usual training days. This system leaves the week end free to spend with one's family, or to enjoy other activities. It has always been my opinion that three days a week are not enough of training for the ambitious body builder or weight lifter who leads and otherwise sedentary life.

If a man works quite hard with the muscles, I would recommend a somewhat different three day training method. One limit day to build strength, for handling heavy weights for a few repetitions under the Heavy and Light System or other form of York Set System. There should be another good training day, working up to at least 12 repetitions, and an easy or tinkering day of training. A man who works hard physically must be careful that he does not make too much demand upon his nerve, he must train without straining, yet gains are made only when demands are made upon the muscles, so he must make demands. We are outlining a method of training which will bring excellent results without too much effort on the part of the trainee. When you make satisfactory gains with one of our suggested training systems, that is a good method to continue. If you don't gain as you desire, change your system, perhaps moderate your efforts for a time, remembering that fewer movements and heavier weights are not tiresome, not as nerve force consuming as working up to higher repetitions. Heavier work builds a surplus of strength, nerve force and energy.

Some men prefer to train 3 times per week, or every other day. The only objection to this method of training is that training comes on a different day each week, on Sunday every two weeks.

The Five Days A Week Training System

Applied to weight training, the 5 day a week training system consists of one very hard or limit day of training, on which you try to equal or surpass your best records of the past, either in weight lifting or in weight training. To succeed you must constantly endeavor to handle more weight, and as you can not work on your nerve every day, we recommend this one day of limit training per week. There should also be two fairly heavy days of training, not quite limit days, but days which make rather heavy demands upon the muscles. One heavy day should see you using 80 to 90% of your limit and practicing at least 10 or 12 repetitions, on the other fairly heavy day you should use 70 to 80% of limit and practice up to 15 repetitions. This latter type of training builds some strength, some muscular size, but most important of all it produces endurance and separation of the muscles. With this 5 day a week training system there should be 2 easy or tinkering days of training. On these easy or tinkering days you use the special appliances which are found in all public gymnasiums, and most home gymnasiums, lots of dumbbell training, Health Boots, wrist roller, head strap, cable or rubber exercisers, Giant Crusher Grips, and others of the result producing and muscle building appliances. These moderate or easy days of training, tone the muscles, keep them ready for the harder days of training to come, build shapeliness and definition. In my own special training efforts during which I made phenomenal gains,

I usually made my hard or limit day of training Saturday. I would rest Friday and Sunday, the day before and the day after the heavy day. Monday would be my 90% day, Wednesday my 80% or 15 repetitions day, Tuesday and Thursday, tinkering days. You can arrange the days in a way which suits your convenience, but this is the way I train the world's championship team and the Olympic team. It has brought world records and world's championships in the past and is the best way to train for the man who is super ambitious.

Irregular Training

This is one of the original York principles which have helped so many to success. It has been partially covered in the 5 days a week training system. The muscles quickly become accustomed to steady work or training, they grow only enough to perform the work demanded of them. If you never used the progressive system, increasing your poundages, your muscles would remain capable only of handling a little more than the starting poundages. That is why workmen, laborers, who do the same work day after day, are seldom strong, why carpenters or bricklayers have only average strength. The muscles become accustomed to doing so much and no more. Finally with advancing years they gradually weaken, and it is harder to do a days work. This stanza of a little poem I wrote at one time covers this true fact about physical training.

If at first you do succeed,

Heavier work is what you need,

For work that does not try your strength,

Will weaken it at length.

Something has to be done to jolt these muscles out of their regular routine. That is where irregular training fits into the body building scheme. It is evident that great or limit demands must at times be made upon the body. This is done on the York Heavy or limit day of training. Rest and moderate training must follow. That is why we advocate the three days a week system, the every other day system, 3! times a week, a 4

40

day training week with two tinkering days and two hard days, or the 5 days a week program with a limit day, two fairly hard days, two easy or tinkering days and two days of rest.

At times to change the structure of stubborn muscles it is necessary to train 3, 4 or even 7 days in succession, and then rest a like period. Surely irregular training is an important way to your physical desires.

Limited Programs

Many men have built weight and strength through very limited programs. They have gained as much as 100 pounds in bodyweight through little more than irregular practice of deep knee bending, coupled with plenty of rest and heavy feeding, particularly the drinking of copious quantities of milk. It has always been the York plan to devise training systems which will cause men to be shapely every pound of the way, York men gain in bodyweight as fast as others, faster in most cases, and have fine physiques and athletic ability with every pound they gain. York men apply the truism, that if you train for strength, shape is sure to follow, and the constant endeavor the handle more and more weight, as we recommend, is sure to result in the acquisition of super strength, and the other benefits which accompany it. Men who follow the York system have gained as much as 100 pounds and become athletic starts of the greatest magnitude. But some men are willing to gain weight at any price, any kind of weight, just so it registers on the scales. This method has been taught in some quarters. While we grant that the practice of a few very heavy exercises, or even one exercise, such as the deep knee bend, will build weight and strength, we wish to warn you that you will not have an attractive or athletic physique if you follow this type of limited program. The minimum of exercises in a limited program should be four or five. Bent over rowing motion, press on bench or standing, abdominal exercises, dead weight lift and deep knee bend, practiced in sets will permit a man to gain weight and strength. But the practice of a limited program of heavy exercises only, will not build for a man a really shapely physique. The exercises listed will bring good results in a minimum of time. Such a program is far better than no program at all, but it will be much better for the aspiring body builder to practice enough exercises to build an outstanding and shapely physique as well as one which is strong and heavy, if that is the paramount desire.

When my time is limited, frequently I will practice three of the exercises of the simplified course, the continuous pull up and press, the high pull up or half snatch, and the deep knee bend and press behind neck. If there is time, I will practice these favorite and result producing exercises in three sets, or nine exercises in all. If I have even less time, I may practice just one exercise a number of times, my favorite of all exercises, the deep knee bend and press behind neck. This one exercise practiced in sets will keep the physique in fine shape for a long period. Any exercise is better than no exercise, so if time is limited, practice the bare minimum of exercises rather than no exercise at all. This one favorite movement of mine can be practiced while shaving and dressing in the morning.

Other Schemes of Progression

To gain in strength and muscle there must be some form of progression. In addition to the double and single progressive systems, there are many other methods of progression. Increasing the weight a count each training day, increasing the poundage every week, or simply increasing the weight as often as you feel your improved condition and strength will permit. When you can properly perform an exercise the desired number of times, increase the weight and continue performing the same number of repetitions.

The York Heavy and Light System

This is one of the original Bob Hoffman training principles which has brought great success to scores of thousands of body builders. To obtain the best results in all around body building, at times the heaviest weights must be employed. It is not possible to practice a full 12 or 15 repetitions with very heavy weights, yet it is necessary to continue a movement long enough to bring the blood to the aid of the working muscle, to supply it with oxygen and glycogen or blood sugar and to remove the waste caused by this effort or combustion. Important gains can not be made without this increased flow of blood or muscle flushing as it is commonly called. With the Heavy and Light System, you select the heaviest weight which will permit 7 or 8 movements. Thus you will not work too often upon your nerve, but the muscles will become big and strong enough to handle very heavy poundages. After a short rest, remove a few pounds of the weight, enough to permit you to practice 7 or 8 more movements with the same weight. Even with the reduced weight as you are somewhat tired from the first set you are still handling a limit poundage. Thus you have performed your limit for 15 movements which you could not do without the Heavy and Light System. Although the York Heavy and Light System is designed for use on your heavy days primarily, it is also applicable to lighter training too, and will bring good results when used in this manner. Some of the most successful York Barbell Men, have used the York Heavy and Light System for long periods in their own intensive training, with marvelous results.

The Compound System

Compound exercises are recommended and included in all York courses. These consist of practicing a series of movements without setting the weight down. Three exercises which involve nearly the same muscle groups are usually selected. For instance, the curl, the back of neck press and the upright rowing motion of the Simplified Barbell Course contained in this book form an excellent compound exercise, or the forward raise, the lateral raise and the front press with dumbbells, or lying on bench, the lateral raise, the pull over and the side swing with dumbbells. The object of practicing compound movements is to keep the blood surging through the working muscles longer, causing them to be better exercised and better nourished. Fatigue is postponed by practicing somewhat different movements. Very good results are obtained with this method of training. Barbells, dumbbells, Health boots, cables, any and all forms of exercising equipment can be used with the compound exercising system.

The York Set System

The York courses were the first regular courses to contain various phases of the set system of training. The set system merely means to repeat the same or similar exercises involving the same muscle group, a number of times. The object of this repetition is to make greater demands upon the muscles. Repeating the same exercise with the set system provides a type or form of stimulation which can not be obtained in any other way. With continued use the muscles will become pumped up with blood, the cells, tissues, and muscular fibers are well flushed or nourished and some of the increased size is retained so that more strength and muscle building results are obtained.

While some of the famous courses were prepared more than 20 years ago, even then the set system was not entirely new, for all advanced barbell users had done considerable training with sets, this may have consisted of repeating their favorite exercise a number of times or practicing repeatedly some particular exercise designed to develop the part of the body they were most anxious to develop.

The York Heavy and Light System already described in this booklet, became a really popular form of set training. With it two sets consisting of 7 or 8 movements each were the accepted practice. It was recognized that at least 15 movements were required to bring the blood rushing to the aid of the working muscle so York set systems included at least this many movements, the 8 and 7 of the Heavy and Light system make 15, the three times 5 with heavy weights are 15, the 5 times 3 with heavier weights are 15, the 5, 4, 3, 2, 1 system, increasing the weight with the same exercise and performing fewer repetitions as the weight is increased, also total 15.

It is not possible to specialize in developing all parts of the body at one time. Most body builders practice from 3 to 5 sets with each movement and if this were done with a course including 12 exercises, there would be 60 movements in all which is too many, except for a few super men who have nothing else to do but train. Therefore we always suggested that a complete course, designed to develop all the major muscle groups of the body be practiced before specializing with sets. In this form of training, the ambitious body builder may perform 3 or 5 sets with 10 to 15 reps, depending upon the exercise, or the desire to gain weight and strength, to lose weight or to gain superior muscular definition.

To gain great strength, 7 or 8 repetitions or less are the usual practice as in the Heavy and Light system, to gain maximum muscular size as well as strength, 10 to 12 movements are practiced in each set, and to reduce bodyweight or gain endurance and muscular definition, 15 movements are included in each set. The fewer repetitions as already outlined, are most frequently used in weight lifting training, but they are applicable to any other heavy exercise if desired. York was the first to use this form of set training, as the usual practice was to endlessly make single attempts in lifting. The York champions by winning hundreds of weight lifting titles proved that the York system is best.

Some body builders are so anxious to train in sets that they use this method always, practice too few exercises and neglect some parts of the body. For that reason we have compiled the many courses in this booklet. Each 12 is arranged so that all the important muscle groups of the body receive attention, each half of the course, each six movements are as complete as possible in themselves. An attempt has been made to include exercises for the most important parts of the body, especially the legs and back. So most any set of six movements if practiced in sets of 3 to 5 will bring good results. As the exercises in each course are arranged in the same sequence, you can easily combine 2 or 3 courses, practicing in turn 2 to 3 series of somewhat similar movements. A simple form of set system was always used in my own training. York courses #1 and #2, practiced together, front curl, back curl, regular press, press behind neck, regular flat back dead lift and stiff legged dead lift, regular flat foot deep knee bend and deep knee bend on toes, bent over rowing motion and upright rowing motion, etc. Two courses combined will bring outstanding results and still leave some time for specialization or training with the many result producing body building devices which are used by the advanced body builder today. Set training is a way to realize your physical desires, but be sure that you practice complete courses frequently, which are designed to develop all the parts of the body so that there will be no weak links in your body. A chain is no stronger than it's weakest link.

Upper and Lower Body Training System

The regular York courses were designed to develop every important muscle group of the body, to bring the maximum of results in a minimum of time with the least expenditure of energy. Each course starts with a curl, a press, a deep knee bend, a pull over, dead weight lift, bench press, side bend, etc. The object being to permit one group of muscles to partially rest while other groups are working. This method saves time and energy. But there are some advanced bodybuilders who have plenty of time and endurance who practice movements only for the upper body one day, for the lower body another day. The object is to keep one set or one part of the body continually flushed with blood, endeavoring to develop these muscles faster. More time and endurance is required with this method of training. We are convinced that an all around training system which involves all the muscles will bring the best results, but the greatest strength is produced, the most muscles developed, the finest physique produced by practicing a wide variety of exercises and varying training systems, so this upper and lower body training system can be included in your training schedule at times with favorable results.

Flushing The Muscles

Throughout the York courses which have been in use for 20 years you will read, when an exercise is continued for a long enough period, usually about 15 repetitions, the blood rushes to the aid of the working muscle. The working muscles need fuel, just as does the engine of your car, so the blood brings the oxygen and the blood sugar to the active muscle. As much as 30 times as much oxygen is transported by the blood during vigorous exercise as when the body is in a quiescent state. This combination of oxygen and glycogen, forms a sort of combustion to provide the motivating power for your every effort. The extra blood surging through or flushing your muscles has often been called the flushing system. It is not a new system, rather it is an old principle used by body builders for many decades. This increased circulation which results from making sufficient demands upon the body, is the chief benefit derived from vigorous training or athletics. This flushing of the muscles and organs activates all muscular and organic processes, feeds all the cells and carries away all the waste. The blood is the only curative agent in your body, the only part that has the power to build, so you can benefit greatly by practicing exercises vigorous enough to cause stimulation of the circulation and the respiration.

After continued action the muscles swell, and usually remain swollen for a considerable period. Some of this swelling is retained, and larger muscles result. All the set systems are based on this long understood and proven fact.

The Overload System

Many men practice with all the weight they can handle every training period. They continually use some form of cheating to overload the muscles, employing very heavy weights and fewer repetitions, taking advantage of various forms of cheating as they exercise. This is a fairly satisfactory form of training if used on the heavy training day only. It will not bring the best all around results, as with the very heavy, limited program previously described, it will build strength, muscle and bodyweight, but not the best looking, best proportioned or best developed physique. Devotees of this overload system habitually use more weight than they can properly handle. Cheat in the curl, using body movement, cheat in every press, using the legs a little, shrugging, leaning forward and bending back, in the rowing motion they use their backs as well as the arms, in the dead weight lift they may use what has been called a hopper, at least bounce the weight from the floor so that they can handle a few more pounds. This method of training has been favored in some quarters but we greatly prefer, except occasionally on the limit day of training, that exercises be performed correctly, and with comparative slowness both in exerting force and returning to the starting position so that the resistance can be felt every inch of the way, and the muscles strengthened throughout.

Big muscles and great strength result from handling heavy weights, and if that is all you want, and you don't care particularly about shapeliness, if you find pleasure, satisfaction or gain fame from handling heavy weights, by all means use the overload or cheating system at times. But if you want to be the best possible all around physical specimen, you should perform the exercises correctly on the vast majority of training days. The author of this treatise actually urges his team members to handle weights so heavy at times in the three lifts that some cheating is required, for this does accustom the body to handling more weight.

Specialization

We suggest that barbell men continue with the York courses just as they are written, for a few months. Year after year these courses produce outstanding men, there is hardly a famous muscle man anywhere in the world who has not laid the foundation for his success with the York courses. After some months of training with the Four Famous York courses, they have gone on to slightly different movements. And it is to avoid the lost time, the misinformation, the improper instruction with it's retarding factors in body building that this volume with it's advanced training methods has been prepared. They are designed so that the man who wants to specialize will specialize properly. We urge you to practice one of the good, well planned, scientifically arranged York courses, two or three times so that the part of the body which is benefited by this exercise will become exceptionally developed.

Another way to specialize is to follow one of the regular York courses just as it is written, and then follow your special training. Should your great desire be to build big, powerful arms, you can practice a large part of the arm course. Should your waist line be less trim, strong or youthful than you desire, or should you be interested in broader shoulders, a deeper chest, or improvement in any other part of your body, you specialize in developing that part using the suggested routines contained in this book. You must be a sculptor, you must mold your own body, look into the mirror, study your physique, see what part is lacking development, or what parts are overdeveloped and plan to bring your physique to a condition of better balance. Take a little off the waist, broaden the shoulders a bit, deepen the chest, slenderize the waist and build a fine set of abdominal muscles. Many of the stars of today were very ordinary in the beginning. This muscle molding we are briefly describing transformed their physiques from the ordinary to the super man class so that they won great honor in physique contests.

The Thousand Exercises

There are 54 exercises in the four famous York courses. In the swing bell course alone there are 48, in the leg course there is 36, in the 4 dumbbell courses 48, in the various simplified courses there are 500 exercises listed. In the "Big Arms" book there are hundreds of arm exercises. In other Hoffman books, hundreds more. In other York courses such as the Leg Developing Course, the Abdominal course, the three expander courses, there are many more exercises. We have tried to offer practically every exercise which will produce it's share of strength, muscle, and super health. Too many exercises can not be practiced in a single day, so keep a record of what you have done. Follow all the exercises in this course over a period of time and you are sure to succeed in a big way.

Advanced Routines

It is wise for the first few months, to follow York courses #1 and #2, exactly as they are written. Thus the foundation of a strong, healthy and well proportioned body will be laid. On this foundation you can build a championship winning body. So take your time, make haste slowly as we often phrase it, give the internal works an opportunity to strengthen and become more efficient so that they can provide for more work and more growth of the body.

As we have said elsewhere in this book, training to keep fit, or build an exceptional body is very simple, the Simplified Course or the Famous York courses which have served well for so many years are what you need. But if you are super ambitious, if you want all the strength and muscle, the finest proportions you can get, a physique contest winning body, you must work hard for it.

By taking your time, by training progressively, by following the correct rules of living, your body should be capable of hard and intensive effort. Many champions train only three times per week, hard and intensively. Such training periods for the man who has the time, the ambition and the endurance may extend for hours. If you had been a visitor to the York Barbell Gym when Farbotnik, Dellinger, Eifferman, Reeves, or Stephan trained here, if you had seen Lauriano, Gri- mek, Bacon, Stanko, and other York champions train, you would have been astounded at the number of exercises they practiced, the repetitions and the poundages. These were all advanced men, men who had won considerable honor and were on the verge of winning even greater honor. When they had nothing to do but concentrate on their training, they trained 5 times per week.

There have been champions of the past who trained two or three times a day, five times per week to reach the heights. Only you can determine which system will be best for you. Only you can tell what is too much, for only you know just how you feel, you must be your own trainer to a great degree. You must follow the other advice we offer in this and other York courses, to constantly strive to handle more and more weight, to make demands on the muscles, and to live right so that nature will make possible rapid building of your body.

The 11 barbell exercises and the 7 dumbbell exercises of York courses #1 and #2 are enough for any beginner, or any person no matter how ambitious who has trained for but a few weeks or months. It is only after a person has made good body building progress that set training should be a part of the program. For little is accomplished unless a good all around program is followed, and the beginner does not have the endurance or the recuperative power to practice too many hard exercises. The beginners do not train in sets, the advanced men do.

We think it best to go into sets gradually. If you are particularly desirous to build some part of the body, or if some part is lacking in development, start improving this part by practicing each exercise twice that is designed for the development of that particular part. For instance, if you want bigger arms, and who doesn't, you practice each arm developing movement in the regular course at least twice. Or you can go through the regular course and then practice many movements for this particular part of the body. That is why with this course, we offer, a dozen good exercises for developing the arms, a dozen good ones for broadening the shoulders, an equal number for improving the mid section or building the chest, special routines for various purposes.

You will get out of exercises, what you put into it. Work hard and intelligently and you are sure to improve in a big way. We offer the best instruction, the encouragement, the know how, the rest is up to you.

24 COMPLETE COURSES
contained in the York Advanced
Method of Weight Training

Course No. 1—The Power Plus Course.

Course No. 2—The Power Course.

Course No. 3—The Weight Lifting Course.

Course No. 4—An Unusual Course.

Course No. 5—An Excellent Heavy Dumbbell Course.

Course No. 6—Leverage Exercises.

Course No. 7—Bob Hoffman's Favorite Barbell Course Simplified Style. Course No. 8—One Heavy Dumbbell Course.

Course No. 9—The Footbell Course.

Course No. 10—Chest Expander System.

Course No. 11—Inclined Board Training Methods.

Course No. 12—Pulley Training.

Course No. 13—Swing Bell Course.

Course No. 14—Mr. America Course.

Course No. 15—Mr. America Course.

Course No. 16—Neck Developing Course.

Course No. 17—Arm Course No. 1 With Barbell.

Course No. 18— Arm Course No. 1 With 5 in 1 Muscle Builder.

Course No. 19—Shoulder Broadening Exercises.

Course No. 20—Chest Developing Course.

Course No. 21—Developing the Upper Back.

Course No. 22—Developing the Lower Back.

Course No. 23—Super Abdominal Course.

Course No. 24—Developing the Upper Legs. Developing the Lower Legs.

COURSE No. 1 THE POWER PLUS COURSE

1.   REGULAR BARBELL CURL. Stand with the feet a comfortable distance apart. Grasp the bar with the undergrip about shoulder width apart. Starting with the arms straight, bar resting against the thighs, curl the weight to the upper chest, lower to the starting position and repeat the desired number of times.

2.   REGULAR BARBELL PRESS. Assume usual starting position, clean the weight to the chest, keeping the legs straight, the body erect, push the weight to arms length overhead. Lower slowly to the chest and repeat the desired number of repetitions.

3.   REGULAR DEAD WEIGHT LIFT. Usual starting position, keeping back flat, raise the bell until you are erect, lean well back at completion of first part of movement. Lower slowly to the starting position and repeat.

4.   BENT ARM PULL OVER. Press the bar to overhead while lying on bench. Allowing the arms to bend slightly at the elbows, lower back of head, return to the starting position and repeat. Inhale as the

weight is lowered, exhale as the weight goes overhead.

5.   SIDE TO SIDE BEND. Place barbell on shoulders, hands wide as bar will permit, feet together. Bend far to right, back to center, to left, to center, and continue for the desired number of counts.

6.   REGULAR FLAT FOOT DEEP KNEE BEND. This exercise is usually performed with the feet a comfortable distance apart, but for better muscle building effect, at times the position of the feet should be varied from close together to quite wide apart. With weight on shoulders, keeping the back flat, go into the lowest possible position, rise to the erect position and repeat. Inhale as you rise, exhale as the body is lowered.

7.   REGULAR ROWING MOTION. Feet a comfortable distance apart, legs straight, body bent at right angles to the legs, bar held with wide grip, the weight is pulled from the low hang to the chest. For variety, the weight can be pulled to the abdomen.

8.   REGULAR PRESS ON BENCH. Usually performed with a very wide grip for best pectoral development effect, it is wise to employ various widths of hand grip at times. Press from chest to over head, lower slowly

to chest and repeat the desired number of counts.

9.　　RAISE ON TOES WITH BARBELL. Place barbell on shoulders. Usually practiced with three positions of the feet, one with heels together, toes out, another with heels out, toes together with feet straight to the front. Greater range of action can be had by placing toes on board. 10 movements in each position is best.

10.　　STRADDLE LIFT. Place a heavy bar between the feet, perpendicular to the front. Bend down with flat back and grasp bar with one hand behind and one front. The exercise is performed by raising and lowering the body over a range of 12 to 18 inches. At times reverse the position of the hands.

11.　　ABDOMINAL RAISE—SIT UP. The simplest way to perform this movement is flat upon the floor with feet under a barbell. Resistance is provided with dumbbell, barbell or barbell plate. Keep legs straight, come up and lean as far forward as possible. The movement is made more difficult and of course builds more strength, vitality and muscle when an inclined bench is used. Sitting sideways upon flat bench or chair, leaning back touching head to floor, while feet are under some heavy object is also a good movement.

12.   BREATHING SQUAT. Performed in a similar manner to #6, one deep breath for the first movement, 2 for the second, 3 for the third, 4 for the fourth, 5 for the fifth, and 5 with every bend after that. Breathe as deeply as you can. Best results are obtained when a breathless condition is created.

COURSE No. 2 THE POWER COURSE

1.   BACK HAND CURL. Similar to Ex. #1, Course #1, except that the upper grip is used. In both forms of curling keep elbows close to the side and make the movement one for the arms only.

2.   PRESS BEHIND NECK. Same position as Ex. #2 of Course #1, except bell is pressed from back of neck.

3.   STIFF LEGGED DEAD WEIGHT LIFT. With a moderate weight stand with heels together, bend from waist until bell touches floor, come erect with back action, lean well back and repeat. With heavier weight it may be wiser to stand with feet a comfortable distance apart to avoid straining the back. One must be careful with this exercise, but it is a very good muscle building movement for those who have flexible backs. Advanced men can usually perform this movement standing on a box, to obtain the longest possible range of action.

4.   REGULAR PULL OVER. Practiced with a moderate weight as a breathing exercise. The weight is moved in an arc with arms straight, from the thighs to back of head.

Breathe deeply as weight goes back of head, exhale as it goes to thighs.

5. SIDE PRESS. Use barbell or dumbbell. Holding the feet 18 inches apart, curl the weight to the shoulder. Then hold the bell with palm to the front, away from shoulder with the forearm perpendicular. Draw the whole arm slightly back, flexing the upper back muscles. Now press the weight to arms length overhead, leaning body to left at the same time. Lower the arm slowly keeping the arm well to rear. If you have lowered the arm correctly, the weight will almost go up itself when you lean the body to the left and press at the same time. Do this exercise in a similar manner with the left hand.

6. DEEP KNEE BEND ON TOES. Bell on shoulders, heels together, toes out, go into a full squat, turning knees well out, keeping body erect. Rise to the starting position and repeat.

7. UPRIGHT ROWING MOTION. Grasp the bar with knuckles front, hands about six inches apart. Stand with the bar against thighs. With only arm and shoulder strength, raise the bell until it touches the mouth. Lower and repeat.

8.   PULL OVER AND PRESS UPON BENCH. Lay on a low bench so that you can reach back and grasp barbell lying on floor, pull up and over to pressing position, press to arms length, lower back of head, pull up and press and continue.

9.   STRADDLE HOP. Bell on back of shoulders, heels together, jump the feet to the side, back to center, to side and continue with a regular cadence for the desired number of counts. High repetitions are the usual plan in this exercise.

10.   BEND   OVER   OR   GOOD MORNING EXERCISE. Stand with feet a comfortable distance apart, place bell on shoulders, keeping legs straight, bend forward until upper body is at right angles to the legs, back to the erect position and continue.

11.   ABDOMINAL   EXERCISE—LEG RAISE. Can be performed on floor, flat bench or inclined abdominal board. Keep legs straight, raise as high as possible, lower and repeat.

12.   LEG PRESS. This is an excellent muscle building movement when heavy weights are used. In all public barbell gymnasiums, a leg press machine will be

found, such a device for home use is moderate in price and a machine offered by the York Barbell Company will serve you well. With this machine it is easy to exercise with 500 pounds or more and very good results will be obtained. Without the leg press machine, a training partner can lift the weight upon your feet, but even this can be dangerous as the weight can get out of balance and fall. Some few stars become skilled at this exercise and learn to place 300 or 400 pounds upon their feet unassisted. They do this by pressing the weight with the arms, then bringing their feet back under the bell so that they get it in the pressing position. Unless you have help, or a leg press machine, you will not be able to handle enough weight to give the legs a good workout.

In leg pressing, the legs should be held wide enough apart that the bar can be lowered to a position near the body, thus increasing the range of action of the exercise.

COURSE No. 3 THE WEIGHT LIFTING COURSE

1.   CLEAN WITHOUT USING LEGS OR BACK. Stand with the feet a comfortable distance apart. Hold the bell with knuckles front, touching thighs. Without using legs and back, with arm and shoulder strength only, pull the weight to the shoulders. Lower and repeat.

2.   CONTINUOUS PULL UP AND PRESS. Starting in the usual dead lift or cleaning position, feet a comfortable distance apart, knuckles front, or over grip, hips low, back flat, pull the weight to the shoulders, press overhead as in Ex. 2 Course #1, lower to chest, then to a position near floor, up, press and continue.

3.   REPETITION SNATCH. Starting in the same position as in the preceding exercise, but with hands somewhat wider apart, pull the bar to chin height at least, then split the feet, one forward, one back, and fix the weight at arms length overhead, bring feet on line and stand erect. Lower the bar to position near the floor and continue to repeat the movement for the desired number of counts.

4.   TWO ARM PUSH. Stand with the feet a comfortable distance apart, left foot

slightly advanced. Hold bell at upper chest, lean forward slightly, and push, continue to lean ever farther back as the weight is pressed overhead. Lower to chest and repeat.

5.   PULL UP TO CHIN. Start in the usual cleaning position. Pull the weight up to chin or forehead level, lower to near floor and continue with the movement.

6.   RAPID, BOUNCING, LEAPING SQUAT. Performed in same position as exercise 6 and 12 Course #1. The different is that you lower the body with a rush, come up with a bounce and leap a few inches in the air. Then down again, bounce, up etc.

7.   UPRIGHT   ROWING—CLOSE GRIP. Same as Exercise #7, Course #2.

8.   PRESS FRONT AND BACK. First press the weight from chest to arms length overhead, lower to back, press overhead, to upper chest, etc. Continue the movement for the desired number of counts.

9.   REPETITION CLEAN. Somewhat similar to exercise #1 of this course, except that the weight employed is heavier, legs and back are used. Start with the usual cleaning, flat back position, pull the weight to the upper chest, lower and repeat.

10.   REPETITION   JERK.   Clean   the barbell as in previous exercise, stand with the feet on a line a comfortable distance apart, holding the back erect, bend the knees sharply and jerk the weight as high as possible, as the weight reaches the highest point, about top of head, split the feet, one fore and one aft, fix the weight overhead, bring the feet back on a line, lower to the chest and continue for the desired number of counts.

11.   DEAD LIFT TO CONTINENTAL POSITION. About 20 to 40% less should be used in this exercise than your dead weight lifting record. The exercise is performed exactly as in the regular dead lift except you keep on pulling to waist height. If you have a continental belt you lift it up to that, otherwise to the height of the navel.

12.   DEEP KNEE BEND AS IN SQUAT CLEANING. Stand with feet farther apart than in the regular clean. If you were to perform the squat clean you would pull up as in the dead lift, squat and catch it on your chest. From this position raise and lower the body as in the regular deep knee bend except that the weight is on the chest. If inexperienced in squat cleaning, pull the bar to the chest as in the regular clean, hold the

elbows high, the feet wide, the back straight and go into the full squat position.

This course #3 is very similar to Course #3 of the Four Famous York Courses. Course #3 has always been the hardest of the York courses and many believe it to be the most result producing, as we have said elsewhere, you get out of exercise what you put into it, and this course #3 will make real demands upon the body. It will build strength and muscle, super health, and develop athletic ability, as it produces many desirable physical qualities. Speed, timing or coordination, balance, judgment of space and distance, endurance, separation or definition of the muscles.

Time spent in practicing this course will bring you a rich reward for your efforts.

COURSE No. 4 AN UNUSUAL COURSE

1.   TWISTING CURL. In performing this exercise the arms work alternately, one coming up as the other lowers. Curl the weight to the shoulders with palms up, keeping the arms close to the body. Then rotate arms as they lower to the original position, the arms going far to the side of the body. The elbow is kept close to the body throughout this entire exercise.

2.   TRICEPS EXERCISE. Dumbbells. Take a dumbbell in each hand, extend them back of head, knuckles up, elbows almost perpendicular. Without moving the elbows, straighten the arms overhead. Lower to original position and repeat.

3.   DEAD LIFT BEHIND BACK— BARBELL. Stand in front of barbell, reach back, grasp barbell with knuckles front, straighten legs and back, pulling bell to the erect position. Lower and repeat.

4.   ONE ARM PULL OVER. Similar to the regular two arm pullover except each arm is exercised separately.

5.   TOE TOUCH WITH DUMBBELL OVERHEAD. Take a single dumbbell,

extend to arms length overhead. Standing with legs well apart, head turned so that you can watch the dumbbell, reach down and touch opposite toe.

6. DEEP KNEE BEND WHILE HOLDING WEIGHT OVERHEAD. This movement is similar to the squat snatch. Take a weight that you can swing or pull to arms length overhead. Stand with the feet about 24 inches apart, grasp the bar with a fairly wide grip, swing or snatch the weight to overhead, go into the full squat position, rise to erect position and continue for the desired number of counts.

7. DUMBBELL—UPRIGHT ROWING. After a week spent practicing this movement with 10x10 movements, the author of this course established his life time record in the two hands snatch. Take a fairly heavy pair of dumbbells, hold them against the thighs with knuckles front, pull them as high as the face with the knuckles remaining up and elbows high. Use only arm and shoulder strength, lower to original position and continue the movement.

8. SUPINE TRICEPS EXERCISE. This movement can be performed either with barbell or dumbbells. It is similar to exercise #2 of this course except that you are lying on

a bench instead of standing. Keeping the elbows high and as stationary as possible, extend the arms to full length overhead. Lower to original position and repeat.

9.   ONE ARM SITTING CURL. Sitting on bench or chair with palm front, curl the dumbbell to the shoulder or upper chest. You can perform the movement as in a standing curl, or you can twist it, curling close to the body.

10.   TWO   DUMBBELL   SWING— LOWER   AS   IN   PRESSING.   In   this movement the bells are swung overhead as in the regular two dumbbells swing, except that bells are swung from outside of thigh, but in lowering the bells you bring them down as in the two dumbbells continuous clean and press. That is lowering the weights to the shoulders and then to the swinging position at side of legs.

11.   SIT   UP—LEG   RAISING—TOE TOUCHING. Lay on the floor on your back. Now keeping arms and legs straight, raise both simultaneously until you are able to touch toes. Your weight is supported by your gluteus maximus as you reach the high spot in this exercise.

12. ONE LEGGED BEND—STEPPING ON BENCH. This exercise can be performed with barbell on shoulders or with a pair of heavy dumbbells. It is similar to walking up stairs two at a time. But it can be done by stepping up on a 24 inch bench just as well. Perform enough movements to feel the exercise.

This course, consisting of little known exercises will add the variety, the developing of muscles from many angles, which results in the greatest strength, the largest muscles and the most shapely physiques. We ask you not to overlook this course, include it in your training at regular intervals, as it will produce strength and muscle at a rapid rate.

COURSE No. 5 AN EXCELLENT HEAVY DUMBBELL COURSE

1.   THUMBS   UP   CURL—TWO DUMBBELLS. Start with dumbbells at side of thighs, perpendicular to the front. Keeping elbows close to the sides, thumbs up, curl the dumbbells to the shoulder. Lower and repeat.

2.   HEAVY—TWO   DUMBBELL PRESS. Clean the dumbbells to the shoulders, with bells perpendicular to the front, press both together, to arms length overhead. For variety hold the bells wider, parallel to the front.

3.   TWO DUMBBELL SWING. Stand with the feet a comfortable distance apart. Start the swing with bells between knees, swing up with straight arms in arm arc overhead, lower in similar manner, well back of legs, and continue the movement.

4.   BENT ARM PULL OVER—TWO DUMBBELLS. Lying upon bench, press the dumbbells to arms length overhead, lower to back of head arms bent slightly and press or pull the bells to arms length again.

5.   SIDE   BEND   WITH   ONE DUMBBELL. This exercise after a little training can be practiced with a heavy

dumbbell. Standing with heels together, lean well to the side, then back to center, to the side, etc. Practice with the other side in similar manner. The bend should be to the side, but for variety you can make a longer bend part front as well as side.

6. DEEP KNEE BEND AND PRESS— TWO DUMBBELLS. Stand with feet fairly wide apart, clean the dumbbells to shoulders, keeping back straight lower into full squat position. Continue the movement the desired number of counts.

7. BENT OVER ROWING—ONE DUMBBELL. Place hand on one knee or preferably a low box or bench. Row with one dumbbell, pulling the bell from near the floor to the shoulder. Perform this exercise with the other arm too.

8. HEAVY DUMBBELL, SUPINE PRESS. Lie upon bench, pull dumbbells to chest, press to arms length overhead. Pressing may be done in several manners, close to body with bells perpendicular to the front, wide grip parallel to the front, wide grip perpendicular to the front, bringing weights in somewhat so that they are directly overhead when arms are straight. All three methods of pressing should be practiced at various times.

9. RAISE ON TOE—ONE DUMBBELL. Can be practiced with feet on the floor, but best results are obtained if toes are placed upon a board or block. This increases the range of action. Practice fifteen to twenty movements with each foot.

10. CONTINUOUS PULL UP AND PRESS—DUMBBELLS. Start with bells perpendicular to the front and at side of feet. Pull the bells to chest and press overhead, lower to chest and repeat the movement the desired number of counts. This is one of the very best movements.

11. SIT UP ON BENCH—DUMBBELL. Holding a dumbbell on chest, sit sideways upon bench, place feet under some heavy object. Lean back until head touches floor, sit up going well forward and continue the movement.

12. DEEP KNEE BEND— DUMBBELLS OVERHEAD. Stand with the feet fairly wide apart. Pull, press or swing the bells to arms length overhead. Holding them there, lower the body into the low squat position. Come erect, and continue the movement.

All the great strong men of the past and present have spent a good portion of their training time with heavy dumbbell exercises. They are essential in physical training. Heavy dumbbells not only build the muscles directly involved in each exercise, but as they are harder to balance than a barbell, all of the muscles get a good workout, for the other muscles serve as balancers, stabilizers and antagonists. The favorite exercise of many of the greats in the strength world, will be found in this heavy dumbbell course.

COURSE No. 6 LEVERAGE EXERCISES

1.   FORWARD   RAISE—BARBELL.
Feet a comfortable distance apart. Grasp the
bell with over grip, bell touching thighs. With
arm and shoulder movement only, raise the
bell in a half circle to arms length overhead.
Lower slowly and repeat the movement.

2.   LATERAL RAISE DUMBBELLS.
Hold a pair of dumbbells at side of thighs,
bells perpendicular to the front. Raise each to
the side in a half circle to overhead. Lower
slowly and repeat the movement.

3.   ALTERNATE   RAISE—
DUMBBELLS. Stand with dumbbells resting
on front of thighs, bells parallel to the front.
Raise the right arm in a half circle forward to
overhead, then raise the left in similar fashion
while   lowering   the   right.   Continue   this
alternate movement for the desired number of
counts.

4.   FORWARD—SIDE—UP—DOWN.
Start with the bells in the same position as in
the previous exercise. Keeping arms straight
raise to shoulder height, extend to sides, raise
overhead, lower in similar fashion to starting
point and continue the movement.

5.   TWO ARM PULL OVER—BENCH. Assume supine position. As this is primarily a breathing exercise, never use much weight in this movement, advanced men find 50 pounds sufficient, grasp the bell with the over grip, extend to back of head. Keeping the arms perfectly straight, raise the bar in a circular movement, continue past the overhead position and on down until the bell touches thighs. As the bell lowers behind head inhale, as it lowers to thighs, exhale. Perform this exercise slowly, breathe very deeply.

6.   LATERAL   RAISE   LYING— BENCH. Weights of moderate poundage should be used as this also is a breathing exercise, Steve Stanko, former world's strongest man, Mr. America and Mr. Universe winner, never used more than a pair of 20's in this movement. Press the bells to arms length, knuckles out, keeping the arms entirely straight, lower to the side. Inhale as weights are lowered, exhale as weights are raised to a position over the body.

7.   SIDE   SWING   LYING—BENCH. Start with dumbbells at side of thighs while lying on a bench, with knuckles in a half circle keeping the bells parallel to the floor, touch bells back of head. Following the same

plan bring bells back to starting position. Continue for the desired number of counts.

8.   BENT OVER, SWING TO SIDE. Stand with the feet a comfortable distance apart. Bend forward so upper body is parallel with floor, arms hanging toward floor, knuckles out. Raise or swing the bells sideways and up past the body, lower to starting position and repeat.

9.   CABLE   PULL   TO   SIDE—KNUCKLES OUT. Extend arms forward at shoulder height, using elastic type of exerciser. Keeping arms straight, pull to side as far as possible, then back to center and repeat. Inhale as the hands go to side, exhale as they come forward.

10.   CABLE   PULL   DOWN—KNUCKLES OUT. Extend arms overhead, knuckles out, pull elastic exerciser down until lower than shoulders, keeping arms straight throughout. Return to starting position and repeat.

11.   CABLE PULL TO SIDE—PALMS OUT. Similar to exercise #9, except that hands are turned the other way.

12.   CABLE   PULL   DOWN—KNUCKLES IN. Similar to #10, except that hands are turned to opposite position.

In this course #6, leveraging exercises, you will find favorite exercisers of many of the great stars of strength and development. The forward raise with barbell has always been a favorite of John Davis, the holder of the world's heavy-weight records, considered to be the world's strongest man. Certainly this movement has had a great deal to do with his pressing and snatching power, which resulted in worlds records. John Grimek, the greatest physical specimen in the world today, never fails to include the alternate raise with heavy dumbbells in his training program. In his opinion it is one of the best. Steve Stanko, U. S. and world's weight lifting champion, winner of the Mr. America and Mr. Universe crown, performed most of his exercise lying upon a bench, a good share of his course is included with Course #6.

COURSE No. 7 BOB HOFFMAN'S FAVORITE BARBELL COURSE

1.   TWO ARMS CURL. Same as exercise #1, course #1.

2.   PRESS BEHIND NECK. Same as exercise #2, course #2. For variation can be performed as a triceps press, holding elbows high, knuckles up, bell back of head, curl or pull the weight to arms length overhead.

3.   UPRIGHT ROWING MOTION. Same as exercise #7, course #2.

4.   SIDE TO SIDE BEND. Same as exercise #5, course #5.

5.   HIGH PULL UP OR HALF SNATCH. Same as exercise #5, course #3.

6.   DEEP KNEE BEND AND PRESS BEHIND NECK. The author's favorite exercise. A movement which strengthens and stretches all the muscles, tendons and ligaments, squares the shoulders, flattens the waist, raises the chest and stimulates the respiration and the circulation. Assume the usual flat foot deep knee bend position with weight on shoulders, lower into the full squat position, come erect and just as the knees straighten press the weight to arms length.

Lower to the back of neck, go into the low position and continue the movement.

7.   STRADDLE HOP. Same as exercise #9, course #2.

8.   CONTINUOUS PULL UP AND PRESS. Same as exercise #2, course #3.

9.   BENT OVER ROWING MOTION. Same as exercise #7, course #1.

10.   TWO HANDS PRESS. Same as exercise #1, course #1. Also wide bench press.

11.   REGULAR DEAD WEIGHT LIFT. Same as exercise #3, course #1.

12.   REGULAR DEEP KNEE BEND. Same as exercise #6, course #1.

The unique feature of this course is it's novel arrangement. The first four exercises are performed with the same poundage, they are good upper body exercises which will produce and strong and nice looking physique. After these first four exercises, weight is added and the next four are practiced. The second four are designed to speed the circulation, increase the respiration, induce perspiration, thus activating the body inside and out, producing internal strength and efficiency and super health. In this series are the exercises which build super health at a rapid rate. The weight is increased again, with exercise #9, for the last series includes power exercises, all a part of the Power Plus course or #1, in this book. Heavy weights can be used in this series, great strength and large muscles will result.

Four men using one barbell can complete this course in twenty minutes. That is 5 minutes actual exercising time, 15 minutes of resting time. This course can be practiced while dressing and shaving in the morning, while reading the paper in the evening, while preparing for bed, while studying. It requires little time and brings wonderful results. It is the most important course in this book and is suitable for all of the family. It is particularly applicable for training of family groups or men or women of different strengths as the Simplex barbell which is adaptable to this course is very easy to adjust. So little time is required to practice this course, that lack of time is no longer an excuse. Only supreme laziness will prevent you from obtaining a maximum of benefit from this wonderful course. Make it a MUST in your business of living. Always practice this full course or a similar one before going on to specialize in developing some special part of the body.

This course originally was made for military training. It can be practiced by the numbers with four men training with each barbell. 10 barbells will suffice for the training of 40 men, and 30 minutes would be ample training for the movements of this course #7, your instructor's favorite, warming up and a neck or abdominal exercise or two. Therefore, the same 10 barbells over a period of time could be used to build the bodies of a great many men. This type of training is ideal for athletic teams and also serves well for any group of students, a class at a gymnasium or a Y.M.C.A.

COURSE No. 8 ONE HEAVY DUMBBELL COURSE

1. TOE TOUCHING, ONE DUMBBELL OVERHEAD. Same as exercise #5 of course #4.

2. BENT OVER BACK HAND CURL. Standing with feet a comfortable distance apart, rest non lifting hand on knee or preferably on low box or bench. Hold bell with knuckles front, bell parallel to the front. Holding elbow as stationary as possible curl the weight up to the gooseneck position of arm. Lower slowly and repeat.

3. BENT OVER REGULAR CURL. Same as exercise #9 of course #4.

4. ONE ARM PULL UP AND PRESS. Same as exercise #10 of course #5, except that only one arm and one dumbbell is used.

5. ONE ARM SWING. Stand with feet a comfortable distance apart. Hold a comparatively heavy dumbbell in one hand between knees, place non lifting hand on other knee, swing the dumbbell well back behind the knees, swing forward and upward in a half circle until bell is overhead, lower and repeat. This movement can be performed a number of repetitions with each hand in

turn, or an exchange can be made between each swing as the bell is about face height.

6.   UPRIGHT ROWING. Same as exercise #7, course #4, except that only one dumbbell is used.

7.   ONE HAND MILITARY PRESS. Standing with feet together, bell is pulled to shoulder. Extending non lifting arm to the side, and maintaining the straight or military position, the bell is pressed to arms length overhead. Holding the erect position greatly reduces the weight which can be used in this exercise. Saxon, who is credited with a bent press of 371, at one time held the worlds record with just 125 in this style of lifting.

8.   ONE HAND SWING AND SPLIT. This movement was at one time a comparative lift and the best performers could handle their bodyweight or more. The movement starts as in exercise #5 of this course, but impetus is given to the bell by swinging farther back, and as the weight reaches the highest point, the lifter suddenly splits his feet fore and aft, as in the two hands snatch, thus fixing the arm overhead. The non lifting hand on the opposite knee and the flat back maintained during the swing and in the performance of this movement. Lower the

bell and continue for the desired number of counts.

9.   ONE HAND SNATCH WITHOUT MOVING FEET. Start with the feet a comfortable distance apart. Assuming the usual cleaning or dead lifting position with flat back and non lifting hand upon the knee, with the dumbbell resting on floor parallel to the front, give a strong pull and bring the dumbbell to arms length overhead. The feet remain stationary but a moderate bending of the knees is permitted as the weight goes overhead. Lower and repeat.

10.   SIDE PRESS. Same as exercise #5 of course #2.

11.   BENT OVER ROWING MOTION. Same as exercise #7 of course #5.

12.   SIDE TO SIDE BEND. Same as exercise #5 of course #5.

This type of training became popular during World War 2. There were restrictions on the use of iron and steel for barbells, so scores of thousands of York barbells were made with concrete weights, which permitted the use of a swingbell but only one dumbbell. A great many body builders received good results from this single dumbbell training, and we felt this one dumbbell course worthy to be included with this book of courses.

COURSE No. 9 THE FOOTBELL COURSE

1. ONE LEG FORWARD RAISE STANDING. Strap on a pair of iron boots. Stand where you can balance the body with hand opposite to the leg being exercised. Keeping leg straight, raise it forward and as high as possible. Lower and repeat.

2. PULLING KNEE HIGH STANDING. Assuming the same position as in exercise #1, this time raise the knee as high as possible to the chest. Lower slowly and repeat. In these single boot exercises, exercise one leg and then the other.

3. PULL UP AND EXTEND. Similar to exercise #2 except that the knee is not pulled quite so high, then the leg is extended straight to the front. Back to raised knee position, lower and repeat.

4. SIDE LEG RAISE. The favorite Footbell or Iron Boot exercise of John Grimek. Starting in the same position as in the other three exercises, keeping the leg straight it is raised as high as possible to the side. In the case of Grimek this means to the height of the head. Lower slowly and repeat.

5.   ONE LEGGED CURL STANDING. Same starting position as the other movements. Keeping knees stationary, the bell is curled with action of the biceps of the thigh, as high as possible. Lower slowly and repeat the desired number of counts.

6.   SITTING, EXTENDING ONE LEG. Sit on the edge of bench, raise the lower leg to that entire leg is straight. Lower slowly and repeat the desired number of counts.

7.   LEG RAISE LYING. This is primarily an abdominal exercise but it also provides muscle building movement for the thighs. Lie on the floor, with hands under buttocks or holding some stationary object back of head. Keeping legs straight, raise the legs up overhead and somewhat back. Lower and repeat.

8.   LEG SPREAD. Bringing the legs overhead as in the former exercise, and keeping them straight, spread as far to the side as possible, back to center the repeat.

9.   LYING ON SIDE—LEG UP AND OVER. Lying on side extend upper leg well back of body raise it and bring it forward until far in front of body. Raise and carry it back to starting position. Repeat the movement the desired number of times.

10.   LEG PRESS OUT LYING. Lay flat on back. Pull legs up until they touch chest, extend to front holding them inches off the floor. Continue the movement the desired number of counts. It is a good leg and abdominal exercise.

11.   INVERTED BICYCLE RIDE. Pull the feet up overhead, so that the body rests on the shoulders and upper back, elbows on hips support the body in this position. Lower one leg, and as the other is lowered push the first leg overhead. Continue with a movement similar to riding a bicycle.

12.   LEG CURL LYING—BOTH LEGS. This movement is usually done with a barbell thrust through the boots, but if desired it can be performed with two boots only. Extend legs out over bench, lay face down, curl the legs up as far as possible, lower and repeat. Some prefer to practice this movement on a slant board at only a slight angle.

It has frequently been said that a man is as old as his legs. With athletes as well as the general public, the legs weaken first, and when legs weaken a man or woman is old. Few people use the legs for anything except to stand on or to walk slowly with, and this provides little exercise for a part of the body. The special exercises included in this course will bring back life to the legs, youthify them, make them strong and flexible. Many athletes past their prime have again become stars through the practice of these movements. The hip girdle is very similar to the shoulder girdle and is capable of a great many movements. To gain bulk, to gain strength, to improve your physique, these Footbell or Health Boot exercises should be made a regular part of your training program.

COURSE No. 10 CHEST EXPANDER SYSTEM

1. FRONT PULL, KNUCKLES UP. While springs or round elastics can be used in practicing these movements, the flat band type of rubber is well liked by the majority. Extend the expander forward to straight arms, knuckles out, keeping arms straight, extend as far as possible to the side at shoulder height, back to front and continue the movement. Breathe in as the expander is stretched, exhale as the hands come back to center.

2. ARCHERS MOVEMENT. Stand with one hand extended, to the side, the other held as in pulling a bow, pull the back hand to the rear until it is straight. Exercise the other arm in a similar manner.

3. FRONT PULL, KNUCKLES IN. Similar to exercise #1 of this course except that the knuckles are turned in throughout the movement.

4. DIAGONAL FRONT PRESS. Hold the expander in front of body one hand up, one down, from this position press out to extended arms. At times reverse the position so that the other hand is up.

5.   FRONT PRESS. Hold hands in front of body at shoulder height, knuckles out, press arms to side.

6.   ONE ARM CURL. Thrust one foot through a handle of the expander. From this position practice the curl with knuckles up and with palm up.

7.   ONE ARM ROW. From the same position as in the preceding exercise, knuckles front, pull up to chin as in upright rowing.

8.   PULL   FROM   ABOVE— KNUCKLES OUT. Extend arms to full length overhead. Keeping knuckles out and arms straight, pull down to shoulder level or below.

9.   PULL   FROM   ABOVE— KNUCKLES IN. Similar to the preceding exercise except that hands are turned with knuckles in.

10.   ONE ARM PRESS. Hold expander behind back, when right hand is pressing, the left hand is held with back of hand against the buttocks. From this position press overhead. Exercise the other arm in turn.

10A. TRICEPS EXERCISE. The expander and the lower hand are in the same position as in exercise ten. The elbow of the working arm is held high, the hand extended to the shoulder, knuckles up. The arm is drawn to full length over head as in performing a similar movement with barbell or dumbbells in other courses of this book.

11.   BACK PRESS. Considered to be one of the best exercises for developing the arms. Place expander behind your back, with hands in such a position that you can press them to the side.

12.   SHOULDER   SPREAD.   This movement is practiced from the arms extended position of the preceding exercise. Keeping arms straight, compress shoulders as much as possible, then spread them as far as you can, trying to spread your shoulders inches farther. This movement will really broaden the shoulders. If you are under 25 you can expect not only a gain in muscular thickness of the deltoids, a stretching and widening of the shoulder attachments, tendons and ligaments, but an actual growth of the shoulder bones, thus making the shoulders much wider.

Exercises performed with springs, rubber or elastics have proven their worth over a period of many years. They will produce a magnificent upper body, broad shoulders, broad back, rounded deep chest, and splendid arms. Years ago when the German weight lifting team, who were then world's champions, visited this country for a contest with our York team, they brought with them heavy rubber cables which they used regularly. Many winners of important physique contests have carried a set of cables with them everywhere they went, used them at every opportunity, and greatly improved their physiques with this form of training. John Farbotnik, Mr. America and Mr. Universe winner, starting with cables alone, built his first extra 15 pounds of muscle with cables. He carried them with him everywhere and he feels that cables played a very important part in helping him win not only his big titles, but special awards of best chest, best back, and best arms as well.

COURSE No. 11 INCLINED BOARD TRAINING METHODS

1.   LATERAL RAISE—LYING. Similar to exercise #6 of course #6, except that inclined board is used instead of flat bench.

2.   DECLINE LATERAL RAISE. Similar to first movement of this course except that head is at the lower end of the abdominal or slant board while this movement is being practiced. It develops the muscles from a different angle and adds to the roundness, and the depth of the chest muscles.

3.   FORWARD RAISE LYING. Starting with a position similar to the thigh position of the two arm pull over, with arms straight, pull the bell up and back in a circular movement.

4.   TRICEPS PRESS. This movement can be performed with barbell or dumbbells, and is similar to exercise #2 of course #4, except that the inclined board placed the muscles in action from a somewhat different position.

5.   FLYING EXERCISE. This movement is somewhat similar to exercise #6 of course #6 except that elbows remain bent

throughout. The movement is similar to that of a bird in flight, and excellent pectoral building results are obtained. Several times as much weight can be used in this movement as in the stiff arm lateral raise lying.

6.　　DECLINE PRESS. This is a little known exercise which has good potentialities for building chest, shoulders and arms. It is similar to the lying press, except that you lay on the decline board, feet raised, head down, and thus exert force and build strength from a different angle.

7.　　TWO ARM CURL—DUMBBELLS. The bells are held with palms up in the regular curl position. Curl from this position until the bells are at chest height.

8.　　TWO ARM WIDE PRESS. This movement is somewhat similar to the flying movement for at the low part of the exercise the bells are held very wide, from this point as they are pressed overhead they come closer together until they nearly touch overhead.

9.　　THUMBS UP CURL AND PRESS. This movement starts from the same position as exercise #7 of this course except that the bells are held perpendicular to the front, thumbs are up throughout the movement.

Curl the bells to the shoulders and then press overhead.

10. TWO ARM PRESS DUMBBELLS — ARMS CLOSE — BELLS PERPENDICULAR TO THE FRONT. Differs from exercise #8, in the fact that the bells are pressed straight up and down from a position with elbows against the body.

11. TWO ARMS ROWING—BARBELL. This movement can be performed either with barbell or dumbbells. Lie face down or prone on the inclined board. If barbell is employed it is drawn up until it touches the under surface of the board. If dumbbells are used they are drawn up well to the side. This movement placed the muscles in action very similarly to the 45 degree rowing position, but lying upon the bench makes the movement strictly a rowing exercise as there is no possibility for using the back or shoulders, thus robbing the exercise of some of its value.

12. TWO ARMS PRESS—BARBELL. A much more difficult exercise than pressing on an ordinary bench, and considerably less weight must be used. It has unusual value in building a high chest.

Winners of important physique contests spend a great deal of their training time with inclined board exercises. For many years this type of training has been practiced by York's Mr. Americas as well as other physique stars who trained here before gaining their greatest triumphs. These exercises are most excellent for building rounded, deep pectorals, in all a very high chest. George Eifferman, Mr. America's winner, is one of the finest examples of this type of training. He excels at the heavy press in this position and has won for himself a set of pectorals, an upper body, that is unsurpassed in muscular development. Pressing in this position has added many pounds to the press record of many international weight lifting stars.

COURSE No. 12 PULLEY TRAINING

1. PULL DOWN STANDING, STRAIGHT ARMS. Face the pulley or 5 in 1 Muscle Builder, keeping arms straight, avoiding body action as much as possible, pull from over head to the thighs.

2. TRICEPS EXERCISE STANDING. Stand facing the pulleys with elbows against side of body. Straighten arms downward with triceps action.

3. LYING CURL. Lying upon floor, if training in a gym, or upon the bench of the 5 in 1 Muscle Builder, curl to the chest. Back of head toward Muscle Builder.

4. PULL DOWN TO THIGHS— LYING. Performed in the same position as preceding exercise, but is done with straight arms. The handle of the pulley is pulled from arms length overhead to the thighs.

5. CURLING TO FOREHEAD— SITTING. Facing the Pulley Machine, curl to the head. Avoid making a rowing movement of this exercise by keeping elbows high and stationary.

6. LATISSIMUS PULL TO FRONT OF NECK—WIDE GRIP. Face the pulley

machine, grasp the pulley bar with the widest possible grip, pull the bar from straight arms over head until it touches the upper chest at the base of the neck.

7. LATISSIMUS PULL TO BACK OF NECK FACING. From same position as in preceding exercise, same hand grip, pull the bar to back of neck or shoulders.

8. LATISSIMUS PULL TO BACK OF NECK TURNED FROM PULLEY MACHINE. Similar to the preceding movement except back is turned to pulley machine, thus bringing different muscles into play.

9. ROWING TO UPPER CHEST— CLOSE GRIP. In rowing with the 5 in 1 Muscle Builder, a good position is to sit on flat bench, feet against uprights of the machine. From this position slightly leaned back, using close grip in this particular movement, pull the bar to chest. Avoid back movement as much as possible, unless you wish to make a back movement of this exercise instead of an arm and shoulder developer.

10. ROWING TO UPPER CHEST— WIDE GRIP. Similar to preceding movement except a much wider grip is used. This hand

position can be varied as desired on different training days.

11. CURL ROWING TO UPPER CHEST. Same general position as #9, except that hands are turned into the curling position with palms up. In this case the elbows are permitted to drop as the bar is brought to chest so it becomes a rowing movement instead of a curl as previously described in exercise 5.

12. PULL DOWN FROM OVERHEAD TO THIGHS. More weight can be used in this movement than others of this result producing series of pulley exercises. The movement is started with arms straight and extended overhead, the pulley bar is pulled down close to the body until it touches the thighs.

Pulley exercises have been practiced for over a hundred years with good results. But it has only been in the last two decades that heavy pulley work has been a part of advanced body building. All the stars of the present spend a good share of their training time at pulley work. Pulleys serve best for developing a broad back, a broad curved latissimus. While they do place the muscles in operation in a different manner than with most weight training exercises, while they do improve all of the upper body, they serve best as back and pectoral developers. All body building gymnasiums have pulleys as a part of their body building equipment, and the man who exercises at home, can not expect the best results without including this 5 in 1 form of training in his program. The pulleys of the 5 in 1 Muscle Builder are excellent for this form of training.

COURSE No. 13 SWING BELL COURSE

1. ROTATING SWING BAR—ARMS STRAIGHT OVERHEAD. With this movement you should make your start with a light weight. With the swing bar overhead, the feet a comfortable distance apart, swing or rotate the body around in a circle. Bend far to the front, then to the side, then far back, then to the other side, continuing the movement by circling the swing bell and the upper body.

2. HIGH PULL UP TO OVERHEAD. Starting with the bell across front of thighs, knuckles front, with arm and shoulder strength alone, pull the swing bell up past the top of head to arms length overhead. The hands are bent and the backs of them are up the entire way.

3. FORWARD RAISE WITHOUT BODY MOVEMENT. Start in the same position as #2. The bell is raised in an arc overhead, arms straight throughout, lower slowly in similar manner and continue the exercise for the desired number of movements.

4. SWING FROM SIDE TO SIDE IN ARC OVERHEAD. Hold the swing bell with

the knuckles front. Turn to the side and bend and twist so that the bell touches or comes near to the floor to the right of the body with the bell perpendicular to the front. Hold the arms as straight as possible as you lift or swing the bell up and over in a huge circle until it touches the floor in a position similar to the starting position but on the other side of the body. Back to starting position and repeat.

5.   SWINGING   WEIGHT   AS   IN TURNING WHEEL. Hold the swingbell in the usual starting position, in front of thighs, knuckles   front.   With   little   or   no   body movement start the bell in a circle toward the left, up and around to the right describing a circular or wheel like movement. Perform a series of exercises to the left and another to the right.

6.   STIFF ARM—FULL BODY SWING. If there were only one movement with a swing bell and it was this exercise, the swing bar would play an important part in building strength, health and muscles with weights. Stand with the feet a comfortable distance apart, the knees are kept straight throughout the movement until the bar approximately touches the floor behind the legs.

Swing the bar up in a half circle, keeping the arms straight throughout. The movement should be performed comparatively slowly to obtain the maximum of muscle building benefit.

7.   TWO   HANDS   SNATCH   AND SPLIT. Similar to exercise #3 of course #3, except that Swing Bell is employed instead of barbell.

8.   SWINGING   EXERCISE—GUN TYPE. The popular gun swinging exercise used to develop the men of our armed forced. A gun weighs a little more than 9 pounds and can not be increased in weight as can the swing bell, so far less benefit is obtained. Start in the usual position of bell, hands and feet, but with the body leaning slightly forward. Swing from this position to the side and overhead, turning the body and rotating on the balls of the feet as the weight goes overhead and to the side, then back to the starting position and movement to a similar position on the other side of the body. When this movement is performed with a regular cadence, a big half circle will be traced from a position overhead on the right to a similar position on the left. With practice and the use of heavier weights you will put your entire body into action with some movement of the

legs and considerable raising and lowering of the body.

9. TRICEPS EXERCISE. Similar to other triceps exercises in this course, those performed with barbell, dumbbells, both standing and lying, with a single dumbbell and with expanders standing. Start this movement in the palms up, curl position, swing the bell up and back of head, holding the elbows high and stationary, pull, or press the bell to arms length.

10. SWING FROM CENTER TO SIDE OVERHEAD. This movement is somewhat similar to exercise #6 of this course. It differs in the fact that instead of merely extending the swing bell overhead, it is lifted or swung up to a position at the right, body twisted so that the bar is perpendicular to the front, then back to the low position at center, and swung with stiff arms and turning body far up to the left. This form of swinging is somewhat similar to the gun swinging type except that it is done with the arms and shoulders and without the movement of the legs and back which are a part of #8.

11. TEETOTUM OR TWISTING DEAD LIFT. Start with the usual position. With the legs as straight as possible, bend and twist to the side so that the bar touches the floor or

ground at the side of the right foot, back to center and then down to a similar position at the left, back to center and continue the movement.

12. COMPOUND SWING BELL EXERCISE. To practice a compound exercise you select any three good movements from this course, and without stopping at the end of the first or second continue until all three are practiced.

COURSE No. 14 MR. AMERICA COURSE

There are so many good exercises, and over a period of time all of them are practiced by the advanced body builder, so it is difficult to select the 12 best. We have endeavored to do this. Nearly all the great physique champions either live in York or trained in York before their greatest triumphs and these exercises are the movements they most generally practiced. You will know when you practice them that you are following the system which made Grimek, Stanko, Bacon, Lauriano, Reeves, Stephen, Dellinger, Eifferman, and Farbotnik great.

1.   ONE ARM SITTING CURL. Exercise #9 or course #4.

2.   WIDE PRESS BENCH—BARBELL. Same as Exercise #8 of course #1, usually practiced with the widest possible hand grip, but variations of hand grips provide additional benefit.

3.   REGULAR DEAD WEIGHT LIFT. Same as Exercise #3 of course #1. Too many advanced body builders have a tendency to be mirror athletes, to practice only movements which develop the most noticeable muscles when looking in a mirror.

In this course we have included some heavy exercises such as the dead weight lift, the regular rowing movement, the raise on toes and the deep knee bend so that the physique star will be very strong and super healthy. A chain is no stronger than its weakest link, the physique star should strive to be strong all over, inside and out.

4.   BENT ARM PULL OVER. Exercise #4 of course #1.

5.   SIDE TO SIDE BEND WITH ONE DUMBBELL. Exercise #5 of course #5.

6.   TRICEPS   EXERCISE STANDING—TWO   DUMBBELLS. Exercise #2, course #4.

7.   REGULAR BENT OVER ROWING MOTION. Exercise #7, course #1.

8.   WIDE PULL DOWN TO BACK OF NECK WITH PULLEYS OR BACK OF NECK CHINNING. Exercise #8, course #12. If pulleys are not available, back of neck chinning will suffice.

9.   RAISE   ON   TOE—ONE DUMBBELL—BOARD OR BLOCK OF WOOD UNDER FOOT. Exercise #9 of course #5.

10.   BACK PRESS AND SHOULDER SPREAD—CABLES. #11 and #12.

11.   LEG   RAISE—INCLINED ABDOMINAL BOARD. Exercise #11, course #2.

12.   REGULAR DEEP KNEE BEND—VARIOUS POSITIONS. Exercise #6, course #1.

COURSE No. 15 MR. AMERICA COURSE

Additional movements.

1.   TWO DUMBBELL CURL SITTING. Inclined bench curl. Inclined bench, thumbs up curl. Alternate curl standing. Regular curl standing. Back hand curl standing. Twisting curl.

2.   WIDE PRESS DUMBBELLS— FLAT BENCH. Incline Bench. Decline press dumbbells or barbell. Regular press, standing. Back of neck press, standing. Pull up and press, 2 dumbbells. Alternate press, dumbbells. Pullover and press on bench.

3.   STIFF LEGGED DEAD LIFT. Straddle lift. Barbell Teetotum. Half snatch. Continen- talling heavy weight.

4.   FLYING MOVEMENT. Lateral, straight arm raise. Regular pull over dumbbells or barbell. Alternate pull over dumbbells. One arm pull over dumbbell. Straight arm lateral. Windmill.

5.   SIDE TO SIDE BEND—BARBELL. Toe touching, weight overhead.

6.   TRICEPS EXERCISE STANDING—1 DUMBBELL. Triceps exercise standing, 1 dumbbell. Triceps

exercise, dumbbells, bench. Triceps exercise, barbell, bench.

7.   HAND ON BOX OR KNEE—ROW WITH ONE DUMBBELL. 45 degree, bent over rowing movement with two dumbbells, alternate, upright rowing, wide grip and close grip. Slow, half snatch.

8.   FIVE IN ONE MUSCLE BUILDER. STIFF ARM PULL DOWN, STANDING. Triceps exercise standing—down pull. Curling to forehead. Straight arm pull down, lying on bench. Curl while lying. Wide pull down to chest.

9.   RAISE   ON   TOES—BARBELL. Three positions, heels together toes very wide, toes together, heels wide, feet straight to front. Straddle hop heavy barbell or light dumbbells. Skipping with barbell. Stair climbing barbell or dumbbells.

10.   CABLES. ONE ARM OVERHEAD TRICEPS. Pull down from overhead, knuckles in, knuckles out. Front pull, front press, back press.

11.   SIT UP INCLINED ABDOMINAL BOARD. Sit up sitting on chair or bench, feet under heavy object. Leg raise while chinning or on parallel bars. Leg twisting and turning

while on bench. Body turning and twisting while on bench.

12.   DEEP KNEE BEND ON TOES. Deep knee bend and press with barbell or dumbbells. One legged bend bench. Breathing squat. Rapid, bouncing, deep knee bend.

All of these movements are in other courses in this book and are familiar to all advanced body builders.

COURSE No. 16 NECK
DEVELOPING COURSE

1.   HAND RESISTANCE EXERCISES.
Placing a hand on each side of the head, force
the head first to the right, then to the left,
resisting with the hand and arm. Place hands
against forehead and resist movement of the
head forward, clasp them over back of head
and resist backward movement of the head,
16 movements each way is a good number.
Resisting in similar manner twist the head far
to the right, back to center, far to the left, etc.
To provide variation place palm of other
hand under chin and force the head up, resist
as it is brought down.

2.   ROLL WITH HEAD ON MAT OR
CUSHION. Place the top of head on a mat or
cushion, so that the body is supported by the
head and the feet. In the beginning part of the
weight of the body can be held with the
hands, but as you become accustomed to the
movement the head will be the main support.
From this position work back and forst, side
to side and roll in a circle.

3.   WRESTLER'S BRIDGE. Lay upon
your back, pull up legs, raise into the
wrestler's bridge position. From this position
you raise and lower. At times you can

support a fair weight, and practice pressing a barbell.

4.   TEETH LIFTING. Most people are under the impression that teeth lifting is only to demonstrate strength, but it really is an ideal exercise to develop the neck and jaw. It keeps the face firm, the neck well developed and causes the entire appearance to be athletic and youthful. At a nominal cost you can obtain a special teeth lifting device and chain which will permit you to practice these fine exercises. Exercises similar to those with head strap are practiced and comparatively heavy lifting is done with the teeth.

5.   WITH HEAD STRAP. With a fairly heavy weight raise and lower head while standing bent over with hands on knees.

6.   WITH HEAD STRAP. With a fairly heavy weight perform a circular motion.

7.   WITH HEAD STRAP. Lying on back on bench, using weight attached to chain, raise and lower head.

8.   WITH FLAT BAND EXPANDER. Loop the expander over the head so that the handles are held in front of head. Pressing the hands and resisting with the head is a good exercise.

The neck is the easiest part of the body to develop, it is also the most conspicuous part of the body when clothed. The practice of neck exercises will improve your physical appearance, making you look very athletic. Strive for a good sized, column like neck.

COURSE No. 17 ARM COURSE NO. 1 WITH BARBELL

1.　　　REGULAR CURL. As exercise #1, course #1, back hand curl as exercise #1, course #2. Regular curl leaning forward with body at right angles to the legs, curl with one hand holding bar with upper grip, the other with palm up. Lying on bench curl barbell from thighs to chest.

2.　　　REGULAR PRESS. As exercise #1, course #1. Press behind neck as exercise #2, course #2. Continental press. Triceps exercise standing, a type of exercise which has been called the French Press.

3.　　　ROWING. Rowing as in exercise #7, course #1. 45 degree rowing assuming a position half way between the bent over rowing motion and the upright rowing motion, row, pulling the bar to the upper chest. Upright rowing as in exercise #7, course #3. Slow half snatch as exercise #5, course #3. Continentalling heavy weight as in exercise #11, course #3. High pull up to arms length overhead, as in exercise #2, course #13 except that barbell is used. Rowing motion behind back, this is a combination shoulder shrug and rowing motion and is performed by lifting the weight to the back of the thighs with knuckles front, and from this position rowing and shrugging as high as possible.

4.　　LYING PRESSES. As in exercise #8, course #1. Performed with very close and very wide grip, and positions in between. Floor press. Same as preceding exercise except performed on floor instead of bench. Pressing from sitting position, press from wrestler's bridge position. Pull over from back of head to chest, and then press to arms length. Triceps exercise as in exercise #8, course #4.

5.　　BENT ARM PULL OVER. Exercise #4, course #1.

6.　　COMBINATION　　EXERCISES. Select any three good arm developing movements and perform them without stopping to rest.

Arm Developing Course With Dumbbells

1.　　REGULAR TWO ARM CURL. Two back hand curl, two arm curl thumbs up, curl under arm pits, extend arms and curl to shoulder, extend to front and curl to shoulders, curl and press, regular and alternate pull up and press. Twisting curl, one arm bent over or sitting curl.

2.   REGULAR PRESS. Alternate press, sitting press, alternate curl and press, side press, bent press. This movement is described in the four York courses.

3.   ROWING. Regular and upright with two dumbbells, bent over alternate row with two dumbbells, one hand row with hand resting on bench or box, one hand half snatch.

4.   DUMBBELLS BENCH PRESS. Dumbbells incline bench, bells close and parallel to the body, bells wide and perpendicular to the body. Alternate press, curl and press. Triceps press, as in exercise #2, course #4.

5.   BENT OVER STIFF ARM SIDE SWING. As in exercise #8, course #6. Bent over triceps exercise. Standing with feet a comfortable distance apart, knuckles back, arms bent slightly, straighten arms to the rear. Hold dumbbells in hand in front of body, twist the dumbbells to the right, to the left and in a circular motion, raise and lower as a wrist exercise.

6.   LIFTING MOVEMENTS. One arm snatch, one arm swing, one arm clean and

jerk, one arm military press, side press, bent press, etc.

COURSE No. 18 ARM COURSE NO. 2 WITH 5 IN 1 MUSCLE BUILDER

1.   TRICEPS EXERCISE STANDING. Exercise #1, course #12.

2.   PULL DOWN FROM OVERHEAD TO THIGHS. Exercise #12, course #12.

3.   ROWING MOVEMENT. Hands in various positions, as in exercises #9, 10, 11 of course #12.

4.   WIDE GRIP—PULL TO BACK OF NECK. As in exercise #6, 7 and 8, course #12.

5.   CURL SITTING AND CURL LYING. Same as exercises #3 and 5, course #12.

6.   VERY WIDE AND CLOSE GRIP. Pull to upper chest as in exercise #6, course #12.

With Special Apparatus

1.   DIPPING ON PARALLEL BARS, with Iron boots to make it progressive. Some advanced barbell men have learned to perform this dipping exercise with nearly three hundred pounds of human weight clinging to their legs.

2.   CABLES. FRONT AND BACK PRESS, rowing and curl, single press, triceps exercise as in exercise #10A, course #10. This performed with the expander behind back, non pressing hand held at buttocks, overhead hand operating in similar fashion to triceps exercise with one dumbbell, two dumbbells, or barbell, standing or lying upon bench.

3.   IRON SHOE—Pulling in variety of ways as specified in course which accompanies this device.

4.   GIANT CRUSHER GRIP. Practicing exercises as included in course which accompanies this device. All Giant Crusher Grip exercises are highly beneficial in developing the arms.

5.   ALL SORTS OF PRESSING AND CURLING With Incline and Decline Board. Practice movements with the incline board which brings the arms into play.

6.   DOORWAY CHINNING BAR, or other bar which permits the same exercises. The Doorway chinning bar has the advantage that it can be mounted high, low or intermediate and permits a wide variety of chinning, dipping and exercises similar to the various pull overs.

COURSE No. 19 SHOULDER BROADENING EXERCISES

1.　　FORWARD　　RAISE　　WITH BARBELL, with dumbbells, alternate forward raise with dumbbells. As in exercise #1, 3, course #6.

2.　　LATERAL RAISE from thighs and from dumbbell touching position behind back, with straight arms to overhead as in exercise #2, course #6. Compound movements of forward and lateral raise.

3.　　CABLES.　　FRONT　　PULL KNUCKLES OUT, same, knuckles in, pull from above knuckles out, and with knuckles in. Shoulder shimmy and shoulder spread. Holding one arm straight to side, one arm straight to front, pull the forward arm to side.

4.　　SIDE　　SWING　　WITH DUMBBELLS—LEANING　　FORWARD. Exercise #8 of course #6.

5.　　TWO HANDS PULL OVER LYING. As in exercise #4, course #2. Two hands pull over and press on bench. If your barbell has high plates you pull it over from a position behind head, to the chest and press, then back to behind head, pull over to chest and continue. Forward raise lying upon back on bench. Start with knuckles up, barbell across thighs, arms straight, raise to overhead keeping arms straight throughout. Lower and repeat.

6.　　MANY　　PULLEY　　EXERCISES WITH 5 IN 1 MUSCLE BUILDER.

7.　　ALL　SWINGING　MOVEMENTS. Notably when they are performed with comparative slowness so that the arms and shoulders perform more of the exertion than the back. One dumbbell swing, two dumbbells swing. Forward swing with barbell, forward raise, with barbells or dumbbells.

8.　　ALL FORMS OF ROWING. With barbells and dumbbells, particularly upright rowing.

9.　　ALL　FORM　OS　SHOULDER SHRUGGING. Heavy regular shrugging with barbell. Rotating shoulder shrug both with barbells and dumbbells. One hand shoulder shrugging with very heavy weight. Shoulder shrugging with bar behind neck.

10.　MANY LIFTING MOVEMENTS. All snatching, pressing, cleaning and jerking. Heavy dead weight lifting.

11. PRESSING MOVEMENTS OF ALL SORTS. As the shoulder plays an important part in all forms of pressing. Military pressing, standing, continental pressing, one arm military, side press and bent press, sitting presses. Flat bench, inclined bench presses of all sorts. Front and back presses with rubbers or springs. One arm press and diagonal presses with elastic exercisers.

12. DIPPING MOVEMENTS OF ALL SORTS. Floor dip, dipping with feet raised, with feet against wall in hand stand position, in regular hand stand position, tiger bends, on parallel bars, dipping on boxes with feet on another box, etc.

COURSE No. 20 CHEST DEVELOPING COURSE

1.   HEAVY LEG EXERCISES. Deep knee bends of all sorts. Approximately half of the muscular bulk of the body is located in the hips and legs, these largest and strongest muscles of the body, those farthest from the heart when in action work the heart and lungs to the limit, as the great need for oxygen is created, the lungs must build greater capacity and the chest is rapidly enlarged. So heavy leg work ranks high as developers of the chest.

2.   ALL SORTS OF DIPPING. Floor, on boxes, parallel bars and hand stands.

3.   GIANT CRUSHER MOVEMENTS. Giant crusher grip exercises are designed to develop the crushing muscles of the body so all these movements are admirable for building the muscles of the chest.

4.   MOST STRAIGHT ARM MOVEMENTS WITH THE 5 IN 1 MUSCLE BUILDER. Straight arm movements pull hard upon the chest, upper back and latissimus and develop these parts rapidly. The chest is not only in the front, but all around, including the sides and back.

5.   PULL OVER AND PRESS ON
BENCH WITH VERY HEAVY WEIGHTS.
A Stanko favorite. Steve Stanko would
employ only a pair of 20 pound dumbbells in
leverage movements lying, but he could pull
over and press on bench a 330 pound barbell.

6.   RAISE WITH WEIGHTS ON BACK.
Lie face down upon the floor with arms
extended in front of head. Keeping body stiff,
raise as high as you can with arm action. This
exercise is made progressive by increasing
the weight of the plate upon the back.

7.   WIDE GRIP BENCH PRESS. All
leading physique stars have exceptional
pectorals and all of them regularly practice
this movement with very heavy weights. The
bench press while excellent for developing
the pectorals, greatly expands the thorax or
rib box too.

8.   DUMBBELL   PRESSING   ON
BENCH. With both wide and close grip.
Particularly the wide press is good, for the
hands move in and out, very wide and the
bells reach the low position, which can be
considerably lower than with barbell, and
close together as the bells go overhead. The
press with elbows close to sides is somewhat
similar to dipping of various sorts.

9.   REGULAR PULL OVER WITH
BARBELL or with dumbbells. Bent arm pull
over with barbell or dumbbells.

10.   PRESSING   BARBELLS   AND
DUMBBELLS on incline and decline bench.

11.   HEAVY FLYING EXERCISES, in
all lying positions with dumbbells.

12.   ALL   SORTS   OF   DUMBBELL
EXERCISES LYING ON BENCH. Lateral
raise, forward raise, pull over, windmill, side
swinging.

COURSE No. 21 DEVELOPING THE UPPER BACK

1.   SHOULDER SHRUGS OF ALL SORTS. Heavy barbell, heavy dumbbells. Shrugging and Rotating. Shrugging behind back.

2.   REGULAR BENT OVER ROWING. 45 degree rowing. Pulling to waist when bent over. Upright rowing with barbells and dumbbells. Heavy lifting such as cleaning, snatching, dead lifting and continentalling the weight to the chest and then the shoulders.

3.   HEAVY LIFTING such as cleaning, snatching, dead weight lifting and continentalling.

4.   PRESSING OF ALL SORTS. With barbells and dumbbells, modified side press, excellent for developing and widening the upper back.

5.   CHIN BEHIND NECK.

6.   DIPPING OF ALL SORTS, PARTICULARLY PARALLEL BAR DIPPING.

7.   MANY CABLE EXERCISES. Pull downs, front and back press, upright rowing, etc.

8.　SIDE　PULL　WITH　CABLES. Knuckles in and knuckles out.

9.　SHOULDER　SHIMMY　AND SHOULDER SPREAD. The shoulder spread is exercise #12, of course #10. The shoulder shimmy is a popular variation of the shoulder spread, for the shoulders are allowed to come back with a jerk in this exercise so that the muscles on the outside of the shoulder blades touch, and then the shoulders are spread with a jerk. The entire movement is done rapidly with a jerking or shimmying effect.

10.　5　IN　1　MUSCLE　BUILDER EXERCISE. Most every exercise which is practiced with this machine develops the upper back, particularly the various rowing motions, and the pull downs from above. The latissimus dorsi muscles provide most of the width to the upper back and these upper side and upper back muscles, impart the breadth and the pleasing curve to the upper back.

11.　WIDE PULL DOWN TO FRONT AND BACK OF NECK, Facing The 5 In 1 Muscle Builder and turned away.

12.　ALL SORTS OF PULL OVERS. The Latissimus Dorsi muscles are designed to pull the straight arm down as in striking a blow with an axe. Pull overs while lying provide similar action and cause development of this muscle, so you know that the constant practice of pull overs of all sorts will develop the upper back.

It's important to develop a broad back. The upper back muscles add to the complete chest measurement, and are very impressive in performing muscle control. To succeed well in physique contests you need the finest back you can develop.

COURSE No. 22 DEVELOPING THE LOWER BACK

1. REGULAR DEAD WEIGHT LIFT. Exercise #3, course #1.

2. STIFF LEGGED DEAD WEIGHT LIFT. Exercise #3, course #2.

3. BARBELL TEETOTUM or twisting dead weight lift. Same as exercise #11, course #13, except that barbell is used instead of swing bell.

4. GOOD MORNING EXERCISE OR BEND OVER. Exercise #10 of course #2.

5. REGULAR TWO HANDS SNATCH. Same as exercise #3 of course #3.

6. REGULAR TWO HANDS CLEAN. Same as exercise #9 of course #3.

7. HALF SNATCH OR HIGH PULL UP. This exercise should at times be performed with a heavy weight and at other times with a weight light enough that it can be performed with comparative slowness so that the weight resistance can be felt every inch of the way. Same as exercise #5, course #7.

8. SWING BELL WITH GUN TYPE EXERCISE. Exercise #8 of course #13.

9.   SWING BELL FROM SIDE OF FOOT TO OVERHEAD. Exercise #4 of course #13.

10.   STIFF ARM BARBELL SWING. Long a favorite with John Davis who holds all the world's weight lifting records in his class, this is a most excellent exercise. It differs from the forward raise in the fact that much of the effort is performed with the back. Arms are kept straight throughout as bell is raised from about knee height to arms length overhead.

11.   1 DUMBBELL SWING. Exercise #5, course #8.

12.   TWO   DUMBBELL   SWING. Exercise #3 of course #5.

COURSE No. 23 SUPER ABDOMINAL COURSE

1.   LEG RAISE. Exercise #11 of course #2.

2.   LYING ON BENCH OR TABLE, keeping legs straight, twist turn and swing the legs. As a wakening up exercise this movement can be performed with good effect in bed. In your training quarters an abdominal board, or a flat bench will serve. Extend the legs over the end of the bench, and swing as briefly described.

3.   SIT UP WITH BARBELL, dumbbell or plate back of head or on chest. Can be performed with abdominal board, flat bench or inclined bench. Similar to exercise #11, course #1.

4.   TWISTING AND TURNING UPPER BODY. With feet held down while lying on a table, bench, abdominal board, flat bench or inclined bench, the object is to sit up at least partially and then twist and turn the body in this position. With a Roman chair, a pair of straps back of knees as we have in the York Barbell Gym, this is a very difficult exercise. Not quite as difficult but still very result producing when the body is permitted to hang over a bench of some sort and the body

raising, twisting and turning movements are practiced.

5.   SIT UP ON BENCH. Same as exercise #11, course #5. Barbell, dumbbell, or plate back of neck can be used for progressive weight resistance, swing bell or plate on chest is also beneficial.

6.   LEG RAISE FROM CHINNING OR PARALLEL BAR POSITION. If you have a pair of parallel bars in your training quarters it is easy to practice this exercise. If you don't have, it will pay you to construct a set for they have much value in body building. Press the body until arms are straight. From this position keeping legs straight raise them as high as possible. Lower slowly and repeat.

7.   CAT STRETCH, OR HINDU NAMASKUR EXERCISE. The worlds oldest exercise. A wonderful movement for stretching, strengthening and keeping the back young, as well as beneficial to the abdominal region. Reach down and place palms of hands upon floor, feet and hands three or four feet apart depending upon your height, keeping arms and legs straight bend down until abdomen touches floor, raise head and bend it far back, now hump the back up like a cat stretching, turn head in as if trying to touch knees with chin. Continue this

movement until tired, 30 or 40 should be possible.

8.   RAISE BODY AND FEET SIMULTANEOUSLY. Touch toes as in exercise #11, course #4.

9.   BICYCLE RIDE. Either without weights, bumping waist hard, or with weight resistance using boots. As in exercise #11, course #9.

10.   THE CRAB. Push up into crab and learn to walk in this position. Lie flat on back on floor. Reach hands up, elbows high, touch palms back of head, pull feet under body, and push up into an inverted or crab position.

11.   PULL IN YOUR WAIST WITH MUSCLE ACTION. Standing erect, draw your abdomen in as far as possible. Repeat as many as 50 times. Learn to perform the vacuum as this is a good exercise for slenderizing the waist and rubbing away internal fat. Exhale all air from lungs, closing nose and throat so that you do not inhale, lift the chest as if you were inhaling. The diaphragm will create a vacuum and pull the waist in to a surprising degree. When once you have mastered this movement it is a valuable exercise and very impressing to those who see you perform the movement.

12. TWIST TURN AND BEND TOUCHING TOE. Stand with feet a comfortable distance apart, extend arms to sides, twist and bend down so that one hand touches a toe, the other is held directly overhead, twist, as you come erect, bend down and touch the other one.

COURSE No. 24 DEVELOPING THE UPPER LEGS

1.   REGULAR DEEP KNEE BEND with feet in various positions. Exercise #6, course #1.

2.   DEEP KNEE BEND ON TOES. Exercise #6, course #2.

3.   RAPID SQUAT. Performed with a bounce and jump as the legs are straightened and the body comes erect. Exercise #6, course #3.

4.   SQUAT WALK WEIGHT ON SHOULDERS. Practice this with no weight on shoulders at first. As the name implies you walk forward while in the full squat position. As you become more accustomed to the movement you can increase the resistance by adding weight to the bar on your shoulders.

5.   ONE LEGGED SQUAT OR STEPPING UP ON BENCH. Exercise #12, course #4.

6.   RUSSIAN TYPE OF DANCE, EXTEND LEGS TO FRONT AND TO THE SIDE. Practice these movements first of all with no weight and then start with light weight and add to it gradually. Men who practice these movements have sensational

leg development. You extend one leg forward, and then with a sort of jumping action bring it back to the squat position and extend the other forward. Practice in a similar manner by thrusting first one and then the other leg to the side.

7.   SIDE LEG RAISE WITH IRON BOOTS OR FOOT BELLS. Exercise #4, course #9.

8.   FORWARD   RAISE,   LEG STRAIGHT, WITH BOOTS. Exercise #1, course #9.

9.   HIGH LEG RAISE. Bending knee and touching chest. Exercise #2, course #9.

10.   ONE LEG CURL STANDING. Exercise #5, of course #9.

11.   BICYCLE RISE WITH BOOTS. Exercise #11, of course #9.

12.   TWO LEGGED CURL. Lying on bench, legs extended over side. Exercise #12, of course #9.

Developing the Lower Legs

1.   RAISE ON TOES WITH BARBELL, feet in three positions. Heels together, toes out, toes together heels out, feet straight to the front.

2. STRADDLE HOP with light dumbbells or heavy barbell.

3. RAISE ON ONE TOE, using block of wood.

4. SKIPPING with weight on shoulders.

5. STAIR CLIMBING with barbell or dumbbells.

6. RUNNING with weights when possible, otherwise stationary running.